T0362119

Precocious and Delayed Puberty Revisited

Editors

PETER A. LEE
JOHN S. FUQUA

ENDOCRINOLOGY AND METABOLISM CLINICS OF NORTH AMERICA

www.endo.theclinics.com

Consulting Editor
ROBERT RAPAPORT

June 2024 • Volume 53 • Number 2

ELSEVIER

1600 John F. Kennedy Boulevard • Suite 1800 • Philadelphia, Pennsylvania, 19103-2899

http://www.theclinics.com

ENDOCRINOLOGY AND METABOLISM CLINICS OF NORTH AMERICA Volume 53, Number 2
June 2024 ISSN 0889-8529, ISBN 978-0-443-12929-2

Editor: Taylor Hayes
Developmental Editor: Saswoti Nath

Endocrinology and Metabolism Clinics of North America (ISSN 0889-8529) is published quarterly by Elsevier Inc., 360 Park Avenue South, New York, NY 10010-1710. Months of issue are March, June, September, and December. Periodicals postage paid at New York, NY and additional mailing offices. Subscription prices are USD 419.00 per year for US individuals, USD 100.00 per year for US students and residents, USD 486.00 per year for Canadian individuals, USD 532.00 per year for international individuals, USD 100.00 per year for Canadian students/residents, and USD 245.00 per year for international students/residents. For institutional access pricing please contact Customer Service via the contact information below. To receive student/resident rate, orders must be accompanied by name of affiliated institution, date of term, and the signature of program/residency coordinator on institution letterhead. Orders will be billed at individual rate until proof of status is received. Foreign air speed delivery is included in all *Clinics* subscription prices. All prices are subject to change without notice. **POSTMASTER:** Send address changes to *Endocrinology and Metabolism Clinics of North America*, Elsevier Health Sciences Division, Subscription Customer Service, 3251 Riverport Lane, Maryland Heights, MO 63043. **Customer Service: Telephone: 1-800-654-2452** (U.S. and Canada); **1-314-447-8871** (outside U.S. and Canada). **Fax: 1-314-447-8029. E-mail: journalscustomerservice-usa@elsevier.com (for print support); journalsonlinesupport-usa@elsevier.com (for online support).**

Reprints. For copies of 100 or more, of articles in this publication, please contact the Commercial Rights Department, Elsevier Inc., 360 Park Avenue South, New York, NY 10010-1710; phone: +1-212-633-3874; fax: +1-212-633-3820; E-mail: reprints@elsevier.com.

Endocrinology and Metabolism Clinics of North America is covered in *MEDLINE/PubMed (Index Medicus)*, *EMBASE/Excerpta Medica, Current Contents/Clinical Medicine, Current Contents/Life Sciences, Science Citation Index, ISI/BIOMED, BIOSIS,* and *Chemical Abstracts.*

Contributors

CONSULTING EDITOR

ROBERT RAPAPORT, MD
Professor of Pediatrics, Emma Elizabeth Sullivan Professor of Pediatric Endocrinology and Diabetes, Icahn School of Medicine at Mount Sinai, Director Emeritus, Division of Pediatric Endocrinology, Diabetes Kravis Children's Hospital at Mount Sinai, New York, New York, USA

EDITORS

PETER A. LEE, MD, PhD
Professor Emeritus, Division of Pediatric Endocrinology, Department of Pediatrics, Penn State School of Medicine, Milton S. Hershey Medical Center, Hershey, Pennsylvania, USA

JOHN S. FUQUA, MD
Professor of Clinical Pediatrics, Division of Pediatric Endocrinology, Indiana University School of Medicine, Indianapolis, Indiana, USA

AUTHORS

NATALIE G. ALLEN, MD
Assistant Professor, Department of Pediatrics, Division of Endocrinology and Diabetes, Penn State Health Milton S. Hershey Medical Center, Penn State Health, Hershey, Pennsylvania, USA

KANTHI BANGALORE KRISHNA, MD
Director, Pediatric Endocrinology Fellowship, Associate Professor of Pediatrics, Division of Pediatric Endocrinology and Diabetes, UPMC Childrens Hospital of Pittsburgh, Pittsburgh, Pennsylvania, USA

ERICA A. EUGSTER, MD
Professor of Pediatrics, Division of Pediatric Endocrinology and Diabetes, Riley Hospital for Children, Indiana University School of Medicine, Indianapolis, Indiana, USA

ELODIE FIOT, MD
Pediatric Endocrinologist, Reference Center for Rare Endocrine Diseases Growth and Development, Robert-Debre University Hospital, Paris, France

JOHN S. FUQUA, MD
Professor of Clinical Pediatrics, Division of Pediatric Endocrinology, Indiana University School of Medicine, Indianapolis, Indiana, USA

CATHERINE M. GORDON, MD, MS
Professor of Pediatrics, USDA/ARS Children's Nutrition Research Center, Baylor College of Medicine, Houston, Texas, USA

JENNIFER HARRINGTON, MBBS, PhD
Assistant Professor, Division of Endocrinology, Women's and Children's Health Network, Faculty of Health and Medical Sciences, University of Adelaide, Adelaide, Australia

PAUL B. KAPLOWITZ, MD, PhD
Professor Emeritus of Pediatrics, Division of Endocrinology, Children's National Hospital, George Washington School of Medicine and Health Sciences, Washington, DC, USA

KAREN O. KLEIN, MD
Clinical Professor of Pediatrics, Division of Pediatric Endocrinology and Diabetes, University of California, Rady Children's Hospital, San Diego, California, USA, Division of Pediatric Endocrinology and Diabetes, University of California, Rady Children's Hospital, San Diego, California, USA

JULIANE LÉGER, MD, PhD
Pediatric Endocrinology, Reference Center for Rare Endocrine Diseases, Growth and Development, Robert-Debre University Hospital, University of Paris City, Faculty of Health, UFR of Medicine, Paris, France

PETER A. LEE, MD, PhD
Professor Emeritus, Division of Pediatric Endocrinology, Department of Pediatrics, Penn State School of Medicine, Milton S. Hershey Medical Center, Hershey, Pennsylvania, USA

LAETITIA MARTINERIE, MD, PhD
Pediatric Endocrinology, Reference Center for Rare Endocrine Diseases, Growth and Development, Robert-Debre University Hospital, University of Paris City, Faculty of Health, UFR of Medicine, University of Paris-Saclay, Inserm, Physiology and Endocrine Pathophysiology, Paris, France

RENÉE ROBILLIARD, DO
Fellow in Pediatric Endocrinology, Division of Pediatric Endocrinology and Diabetes, Hasbro Children's Hospital, Warren Alpert Medical School of Brown University, Providence, Rhode Island, USA

LAWRENCE A. SILVERMAN, MD
Pediatric Endocrinologist, Division of Pediatric Endocrinology, Goryeb Children's Hospital, Atlantic Health System, Morristown, New Jersey, USA

LISA SWARTZ TOPOR, MD, MMSc
Professor of Pediatrics, Division of Pediatric Endocrinology and Diabetes, Hasbro Children's Hospital, Warren Alpert Medical School of Brown University, Providence, Rhode Island, USA

SELMA F. WITCHEL, MD
Professor Emerita, Division of Pediatric Endocrinology and Diabetes, Department of Pediatrics, UPMC Children's Hospital of Pittsburgh, University of Pittsburgh, Pittsburgh, Pennsylvania, USA, Division of Pediatric Endocrinology and Diabetes, Department of Pediatrics, UPMC Children's Hospital of Pittsburgh, University of Pittsburgh, Pittsburgh, Pennsylvania, USA

SVETLANA A. YATSENKO, MD
Professor, Departments of Pathology, and Obstetrics, Gynecology and Reproductive Sciences, University of Pittsburgh, Magee-Womens Research Institute, Pittsburgh, Pennsylvania, USA

Contents

Puberty is characterized by gonadarche and adrenarche. Gonadarche represents the reactivation of the hypothalamic-pituitary-gonadal axis with increased gonadotropin-releasing hormone, luteinizing hormone, and follicle-stimulating hormone secretion following the quiescence during childhood. Pubarche is the development of pubic hair, axillary hair, apocrine odor reflecting the onset of pubertal adrenal maturation known as adrenarche. A detailed understanding of these pubertal processes will help clarify relationships between the timing of the onset of puberty and cardiovascular, metabolic, and reproductive outcomes in adulthood. The onset of gonadarche is influenced by neuroendocrine signals, genetic variants, metabolic factors, and environmental elements.

Breast development in a girl 3 years of age or younger is a commonly encountered scenario. Nearly all of these cases will either regress or fail to progress during follow-up, confirming a diagnosis of premature thelarche (PT). Studies show that these girls will have onset of true puberty and menses at a normal age. The authors present evidence that laboratory testing, particularly basal and gonadotropin hormone-releasing hormone –stimulated gonadotropin levels, will show overlap between girls with PT and the rare patients with the onset of central precocious puberty before age 3, mainly of whom have hypothalamic hamartomas.

Premature pubarche (PP) is a common and usually benign variant of normal puberty most often seen in 5-year-old to 9-year-old children. Some providers routinely order laboratory testing and a bone age to try to rule out other diagnoses including nonclassic congenital adrenal hyperplasia and gonadal or adrenal tumors. I review the natural history of PP and studies which suggest that without clinical features such as rapid growth and progression or genital enlargement, it is unlikely that a treatable condition will be found. Therefore it is recommended that patients with PP not undergo testing unless there are red flags at the time of the initial visit.

extensive differential diagnosis includes congenital and acquired causes. Presenting features depend on which class of sex steroids is involved, and diagnosis rests on hormonal and, if indicated, imaging and/or genetic studies. Effective treatment exists for nearly all causes of PPP. Ongoing research will advance our therapeutic armamentarium and understanding of the pathophysiologic basis of these conditions.

Constitutional delay of growth and puberty (CDGP) is the most common cause of delayed puberty in both male and female individuals. This article reviews the causes of delayed puberty focusing on CDGP, including new advances in the understanding of the genetics underpinning CDGP, a clinical approach to discriminating CDGP from other causes of delayed puberty, outcomes, as well as current and potential emerging management options.

Delayed puberty is defined as absent testicular enlargement in boys or breast development in girls at an age that is 2 to 2.5 SDS later than the mean age at which these events occur in the population (traditionally, 14 years in boys and 13 years in girls). One cause of delayed/absent puberty is hypogonadotropic hypogonadism (HH), which refers to inadequate hypothalamic/pituitary function leading to deficient production of sex steroids in males and females. Individuals with HH typically have normal gonads, and thus HH differs from hypergonadotropic hypogonadism, which is associated with primary gonadal insufficiency.

This review focuses on primary amenorrhea and primary/premature ovarian insufficiency due to hypergonadotropic hypogonadism. Following a thoughtful, thorough evaluation, a diagnosis can usually be discerned. Pubertal induction and ongoing estrogen replacement therapy are often necessary. Shared decision-making involving the patient, family, and healthcare team can empower the young person and family to successfully thrive with these chronic conditions.

Managing patients unable to produce sex steroids using gonadotropins to mimic minipuberty in hypogonadotropic hypogonadism, or sex steroids in patients with Klinefelter or Turner syndrome, is promising. There is a need to pursue research in this area, with large prospective cohorts and long-term data before these treatments can be routinely considered.

ENDOCRINOLOGY AND METABOLISM CLINICS OF NORTH AMERICA

SERIES OF RELATED INTEREST

Medical Clinics
https://www.medical.theclinics.com
Primary Care: Clinics in Office Practice
https://www.primarycare.theclinics.com/

VISIT THE CLINICS ONLINE!
Access your subscription at:
www.theclinics.com

Foreword

Precocious and Delayed Puberty Revisited

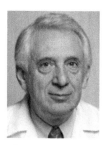

Robert Rapaport, MD
Consulting Editor

The subject of puberty has traditionally been fraught with questions and controversies among endocrinologists, gynecologists, pediatricians, internists, and parents in large part fueled by insufficient reproducible data. The controversies concern theories about the onset of normal puberty as well as etiologies of variations of pubertal development, both early and late onset of puberty. The correct recognition as well as management of these disorders has generated a great deal of interest resulting in novel investigations over the past decade. I am therefore particularly pleased to have world-renowned experts in the field of puberty contribute to this issue of the *Endocrinology and Metabolism Clinics of North America*. The starting article reviews the newest theories explaining the onset of normal puberty. Early puberty events, such as the development of pubic hair, breast development, vaginal bleeding, or complete central puberty, are addressed along with the latest evidence-based developments in their diagnoses, treatment, and outcomes. Partial, incomplete, complete, peripheral, and central pubertal variations in both male and female patients are addressed. Late onset of puberty, including those related to hypogonadotropic hypogonadism, and early cessation of puberty, such as ovarian failure and primary amenorrhea, are expertly examined. Controversial early treatment during infancy of patients with pubertal disorders is also discussed. Finally, guidelines for a practical approach to pubertal abnormalities are summarized. This issue of the *Endocrinology and Metabolism Clinics of North America* will serve as a useful primer for all involved in the care of children with pubertal abnormalities.

Endocrinol Metab Clin N Am 53 (2024) ix–x
https://doi.org/10.1016/j.ecl.2024.03.001
endo.theclinics.com

DISCLOSURE

The author has no conflicts of interest to disclose.

Robert Rapaport, MD
Icahn School of Medicine at Mount Sinai
Division of Pediatric Endocrinology Diabetes
Kravis Children's Hospital at Mount Sinai
New York, NY 10029, USA

E-mail address:
robert.rapaport@mountsinai.org

Preface

Abnormal Puberty Revisited: A Practical Approach

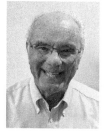 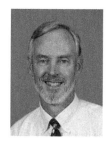

Peter A. Lee, MD, PhD   John S. Fuqua, MD
Editors

Given the prevalence of issues related to puberty in the public and social media as well as newer research findings, it is an appropriate time to review the ways pubertal changes may present at any age. Appropriate management of these children often involves follow-up clinical assessment with varying and sometimes minimal requirements for laboratory assessment, especially at initial presentation. Thus, this issue of *Endocrinology and Metabolism Clinics of North America* aims to present a practical approach to children presenting with findings of early or late pubertal development. After an initial article describing multiple aspects of normal puberty, subsequent articles provide a reasonable approach to patients presenting with evidence of partial or complete early or late puberty. Concerns about early development include isolated breast development or isolated vaginal bleeding before 7 years of age and early sexual hair development. Other aspects of early-onset puberty include the diagnosis of central precocious puberty and the efficacy, safety, and outcome of treatment with gonadotropin-releasing hormone analogues or antagonists. We also include an article regarding peripheral causes of precocious puberty. Three articles discuss key aspects of adolescents presenting with delayed or absent pubertal development, including constitutional delay, hypogonadotropic hypogonadism, and primary amenorrhea. The final article discusses "nontraditional" hormonal therapy during infancy or early childhood, such as induction of the "minipuberty" in known hypogonadal infants.

Endocrinol Metab Clin N Am 53 (2024) xi–xii
https://doi.org/10.1016/j.ecl.2024.03.002
0889-8529/24/© 2024 Published by Elsevier Inc.

endo.theclinics.com

DISCLOSURES

The authors have no conflicts of interest to disclose.

Peter A. Lee, MD, PhD
Division of Pediatric Endocrinology
Penn State College of Medicine
12 Briarcrest Circle
Hershey, PA 17033, USA

John S. Fuqua, MD
Division of Pediatric Endocrinology
Indiana University School of Medicine
705 Riley Hospital Drive
Room 5960
Indianapolis, IN 46202, USA

E-mail addresses:
plee@pennstatehealth.psu.edu (P.A. Lee)
jsfuqua@iu.edu (J.S. Fuqua)

Normal Puberty

Kanthi Bangalore Krishna, MD*, Selma F. Witchel, MD

KEYWORDS

- Luteinizing hormone • Follicle-stimulating hormone • Gonadarche • Puberty
- Gonadotropin-releasing hormone • Kisspeptin-neurokinin B-dynorphin neurons

KEY POINTS

- Puberty is characterized by gonadarche and adrenarche.
- Gonadarche represents the reactivation of the hypothalamic-pituitary-gonadal axis with increased gonadotropin-releasing hormone, luteinizing hormone, and follicle-stimulating hormone secretion following the quiescence during childhood.
- Pubarche is the development of pubic hair, axillary hair, apocrine odor reflecting the onset of pubertal adrenal maturation known as adrenarche.
- A detailed understanding of these pubertal processes will help clarify relationships between the timing of onset of puberty and cardiovascular, metabolic, and reproductive outcomes in adulthood.
- The onset of gonadarche is influenced by neuroendocrine signals, genetic variants, metabolic factors, and environmental elements.

INTRODUCTION

Puberty is the process through which reproductive competence is achieved.[1] Since ancient times, the importance of pubertal development has been recognized. Castration of animals and humans was known to interfere with the development of secondary sex characteristics and fertility. Indeed, some earlier cultures deliberately castrated men to create eunuchs to work with royalty, government, and religious institutions. Previously (and persisting in some cultures today), women were considered to be dangerous due to menstruation and menstrual blood; menstruating women were deliberately isolated. Subsequently, investigators during the twentieth century established the interrelationships of the hypothalamic-pituitary-gonadal (HPG) axis, isolated the various sex steroids, and discovered the necessity of pulsatile hormone secretion.[2,3]

Division of Pediatric Endocrinology and Diabetes, UPMC Childrens Hospital of Pittsburgh, Pittsburgh, PA, USA
* Corresponding author. UPMC Childrens Hospital of Pittsburgh, 4401 Penn Avenue, Pittsburgh, PA 15224.
E-mail address: bangalorekrishnak2@upmc.edu

Endocrinol Metab Clin N Am 53 (2024) 183–194
https://doi.org/10.1016/j.ecl.2024.01.001
0889-8529/24/© 2024 Elsevier Inc. All rights reserved.
endo.theclinics.com

Genetic attributes, neuroendocrine interactions, and gonadal composition influence the onset and progression of puberty. Twin studies have established that the timing of puberty is highly heritable. The sex chromosome constitution of the embryo, XX or XY, determines whether the undifferentiated primordial gonads develop into ovaries or testes, respectively. By 5 to 6 weeks after conception, primordial germ cells migrate into the genital ridge. The environment of the developing gonads launches the developmental pathway directing primordial germ cells to eventually become oocytes or spermatogonia. Eventually, gonadal differentiation, whether ovary or testis, directs an individual's pubertal maturation archetype. During the transition from childhood to adulthood, children typically demonstrate a predictable sequence of hormonal and physical changes. Within the typical chronologic age ranges for pubertal development, individual variations regarding age at onset and tempo of pubertal development occur. Notably, in addition to genetic elements, metabolic, nutritional, environmental, ethnic, geographic, and economic factors influence the onset and tempo of pubertal development.[4]

GONADARCHE

Human puberty is characterized by 2 discrete physiologic processes, gonadarche and adrenarche. Gonadarche denotes the reactivation of the hypothalamic gonadotropin-releasing hormone (GnRH) pulse generator characterized by increased pulsatile secretion of GnRH from the hypothalamus. Increased pulsatile GnRH secretion promotes pulsatile pituitary gonadotropin secretion which, in turn, stimulates the growth and maturation of the gonads accompanied by rising gonadal sex steroid secretion. Hence, HPG axis activity is fundamental to gonadarche, reproductive maturation, and fertility.

Gonadal sex steroids promote secondary sex characteristic development. In girls, increased gonadotropin secretion, luteinizing hormone (LH) and follicle-stimulating hormone (FSH), leads to increased ovarian estrogen secretion causing breast development, cornification of the vaginal mucosa, and uterine growth. In boys, increased LH and FSH secretion promotes increased testicular volume and testosterone secretion. This increased HPG axis activity culminates in folliculogenesis, ovulation, and menses in girls and spermatogenesis in boys.

Following the increased activity during the first few months of life known as the mini-puberty of infancy (see the following sections), the HPG axis becomes quiescent until increased pulsatile GnRH secretion launches the onset of gonadarche. Stimulatory and inhibitory impulses from higher hypothalamic and brain regions modulate hypothalamic GnRH secretion at the median eminence followed by transport through the pituitary portal blood system to the anterior pituitary gonadotroph cells. Acting on its cognate receptor, the GnRH receptor, GnRH stimulates gonadotropin secretion. The pituitary gonadotroph cells synthesize and secrete both LH and FSH. LH and FSH are glycoproteins with identical alpha subunits and distinct beta subunits that confer hormone specificity. Each GnRH pulse is intimately associated with a subsequent LH pulse. Pulse frequency is relatively constant in men with approximately 1 pulse every 90 to 120 minutes. In women, pulse frequency varies across the menstrual cycle with about 1 pulse per hour during the follicular phase and 1 pulse every 180 minutes during the luteal phase.

The hypothalamic GnRH-secreting neurons are physically located within a network of neurons secreting 3 neuropeptides: kisspeptin, neurokinin B, and dynorphin. These neurons, labeled the kisspeptin-neurokinin B-dynorphin (KNDy) neurons, are located in close proximity to glial cells such as tanycytes, astrocytes, and ependymal cells.

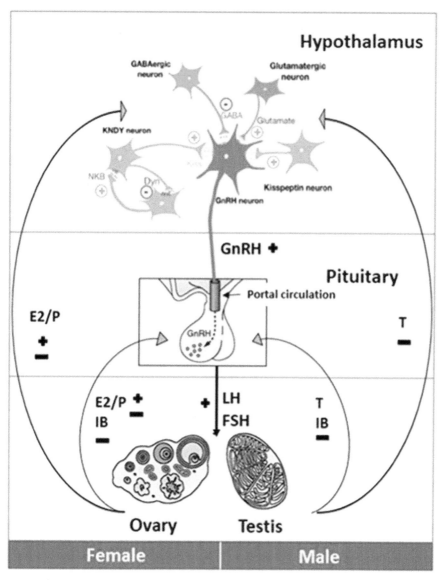

Fig. 1. Schematic representation of the hypothalamic-pituitary-gonadal axis. Kisspeptin, neurokinin B, and dynorphin along with other upstream signals govern hypothalamic GnRH neuron function. GnRH is secreted into the median eminence and travels via the pituitary portal circulation to the anterior pituitary where it stimulates LH and FSH production. These gonadotropins stimulate gonadal sex steroid secretion. Sex steroids provide a mix of negative and positive feedback on the pituitary and hypothalamus. IB provides negative feedback on the pituitary. Key: −, negative feedback; +, positive feedback. FSH, follicle-stimulating hormone; GnRH, gonadotropin-releasing hormone; IB, inhibin B; LH, luteinizing hormone. (Reprinted with permission: Howard SR. Interpretation of reproductive hormones before, during and after the pubertal transition-Identifying health and disordered puberty. Clin Endocrinol (Oxf). 2021;95:702-15. https://doi.org/10.1111/cen.14578. PMID: 34368982.)

Kisspeptin and neurokinin B appear to play major roles in GnRH secretion (**Fig. 1**). The KNDy neurons in the infundibular nucleus in the hypothalamus appear to comprise the major elements of the GnRH pulse generator. For more detailed discussion of the KNDy neurons, the reader is referred to another publication.[5]

PUBARCHE AND ADRENARCHE

Pubarche describes the physical development of pubic hair accompanied by increased apocrine body odor, acne, and axillary hair. Pubarche is the physical manifestation of adrenarche. Adrenarche, defined by rising dehydroepiandrosterone (DHEA) sulfate (DHEAS) concentrations, is characterized by increased secretion of C-19 steroids from the zona reticularis of the adrenal cortex. These C-19 steroids are categorized as "adrenal androgens" although binding to the androgen receptor is limited. These hormones include DHEA, DHEAS, androstenedione, testosterone, and the 11-oxyandrogens. Adrenarche may be evident prior to the onset of breast development in girls and testicular enlargement in boys.

The 11-oxyandrogens, 11β-hydroxyandrostenedione (11OHA4), and 11β-hydroxy-testosterone (11OHT) are formed from androstenedione and testosterone in the adrenal cortex following 11β-hydroxylation by the enzyme 11β-hydroxylase. Extra-adrenal oxidation of 11OHA4 via 11β-hydroxysteroid dehydrogenase type 2 generates 11-ketoandrostenedione which serves as a substrate for reduction by aldo-keto reductase 1C3, yielding the active androgen 11-ketotestosterone (11 KT). Indeed, 11 KT appears to be the dominant bioactive androgen during both normal and premature adrenarche.[6] Longitudinal tracking of a small cohort of normal children demonstrated that 11OHA, 11 KT, and 11OHT increase across puberty.[7]

Despite expanded knowledge regarding adrenal physiology, the etiology for adrenarche remains unclear. Based on urinary steroid hormone profiling, adrenarche may be a gradual process beginning earlier than previously believed.[8]

SECONDARY SEX CHARACTERISTICS ASSOCIATED WITH PUBERTY

In the 1960s, Tanner and colleagues[9,10] followed the physical features associated with pubertal development of children living in an orphanage in the United Kingdom. They categorized puberty into 5 stages with stage 1 being prepubertal and stage 5 representing adult development. For girls, Tanner staging is used to describe breast and pubic hair development. For boys, Tanner staging is used to describe testicular volume, penile development, and pubic hair development. Tanner and his colleagues[9,10] also reported that the tempo of puberty varied between individuals. In general, breast development in girls and testicular enlargement in boys precede pubic hair development. The tempo for pubic hair development is faster such that genital and pubic hair development is synchronized during the later stages of puberty. Nevertheless, discordance between gonadarche and adrenarche may be evident in normal development.

Girls

For girls, increased ovarian estrogen secretion promotes breast development. The development of breast buds with increased areolar diameter is considered to be stage 2; greater enlargement of the breasts occurs in stage 3, accompanied by increased pigmentation of the areolae and nipples. During stage 4, the areolae are mounded above the breast tissue. Recession of the areola to the general breast contour represents breast stage 5. Estrogen also induces cornification of the vaginal mucosa, uterine growth, and acquisition of an adult female body habitus. Palpation of the breast is essential to differentiate between breast tissue and lipomastia.

Menarche typically follows an anovulatory cycle and generally occurs 2 to 3 years after the onset of breast development. During the first year post-menarche, irregular menstrual cycles are common; cycles are typically 21 to 45 days. By 3 years post-menarche, cycles are typically 21 to 35 days. Lack of menses by 3 years post-thelarche or cycles greater than 90 days is abnormal and warrants further evaluation.

For girls, development of pigmented coarse hairs along the labia majora is classified as pubic hair stage 2. During pubic hair stage 3, the hair becomes darker and coarser spreading over the pubic symphysis. Tanner stage 4 pubic hair development is characterized by an inverse triangle spreading to the medial aspects of the thighs for Tanner stage 5. Apocrine odor may precede or accompany the development of pubic hair. Associated findings include axillary hair, acne, and oiliness of the skin and hair. The pubertal growth spurt normally occurs concomitantly with the onset of breast development peaking during mid-puberty with only 4 to 6 cm of linear growth occurring after menarche.

Boys

For boys, increasing testicular and adrenal androgen secretion contributes to the development of secondary sex characteristics. To assess testicular volume, palpation or orchidometer use is essential. At stage 2, the testes are approximately 4 to 5 mL in volume with the longest axis being approximately 2.5 cm. The volume of the mature human testis is approximately 20 to 25 mL. At genital stage 3, further growth of the testes has occurred; the length and diameter of the penis has increased. Spermatozoa (spermaturia) can be found in early morning urine samples beginning during genital stage 3. Nocturnal sperm emissions may also begin around this time. At genital stage 4, penile size has increased, and the scrotal skin has become darkened.

In boys, pubic hair stage 2 consists of sparse pigmented hair at the base of the penis. For pubic hair stage 3, the hair is longer, darker, and extends over the junction of the pubic bones. For pubic hair stage 4, the extent of hair has increased, but has not yet achieved the adult male escutcheon typical of stage 5. Additional secondary sexual characteristics in boys include axillary hair, increased size of the larynx, deepening of the voice, increased bone mass, and increased muscle strength. Terminal hair begins to develop in androgen-dependent regions on the face and trunk approximately 3 years after the appearance of pubic hair. Timing, density, and distribution of facial and body hair vary considerably.

Approximately 50% of normal boys experience gynecomastia, usually in mid-puberty. This is attributed to the ratio of circulating concentrations of estradiol to testosterone being relatively high. In most instances, gynecomastia resolves spontaneously by 16 years of age.

Voice break is another marker of pubertal progression in boys. Among healthy Danish boys, voice break occurred at the mean age of 13.6 years and was moderately correlated with other male pubertal milestones including testicular enlargement, axillary odor, pubarche, axillary hair, and peak height velocity.[11] The pubertal growth spurt in boys, with an average height velocity of 9.5 cm per year, occurs around the end of Tanner genital stage 3 and the beginning of Tanner stage 4.

ONTOGENY OF GONADOTROPIN-RELEASING HORMONE NEURONS

Gonadarche and reproductive competence depend on GnRH neuron development. In the human fetus, GnRH neurons initially develop in the olfactory placode outside the central nervous system. Subsequent influence of growth factors, adhesion molecules, and diffusible guidance cues (both attractive and repulsive) direct the migration of the GnRH neurons. During this migration, the GnRH neurons are accompanied by olfactory-derived axons, olfactory epithelial sheath cells, and blood vessels toward the cribriform plate. Upon reaching the hypothalamus, the GnRH neurons disperse to their final locations, sending projections to the median eminence to release GnRH into the hypophyseal portal vasculature.[12] The precise origin and particular factors responsible for the specification and differentiation of GnRH neuron precursors remain enigmatic. Investigation of genetic variants associated with disordered puberty has provided insights regarding the development of human GnRH neurons. The anosmia/hyposmia phenotype of some genetic variants associated with congenital hypogonadotropic hypogonadism (CHH) reflects the close associations of the developing olfactory system and GnRH neurons. Normal function of the HPG axis is ultimately dependent on the meticulous spatio-temporal orchestration of the migration and function of the GnRH neurons.

MINIPUBERTY

With the availability of more sensitive hormone assays, Forest and colleagues[13] described a transient period of increased HPG axis activity in early infancy. Following the low gonadotropin concentrations at birth, gonadotropin concentrations were found to rise in both boys and girls within weeks of birth. This transient gonadotropin secretion has been labeled "minipuberty." In the immediate neonatal period, low gonadotropin concentrations are attributed to hypothalamic-pituitary suppression by placental estrogen secretion. Upon interruption of placental estrogen exposure, gonadotropin secretion increases.

Over the first few years of life, sexual dimorphism in gonadotropin concentrations has been noted. Boys have higher LH concentrations than girls; LH concentration typically peak between 2 and 10 weeks of age and decline by 4 to 6 months of age. Testicular testosterone secretion occurs with testosterone concentrations typically peaking around 1 month of age followed by a decline to prepubertal concentrations by 7 to 12 months of age.

Girls have higher FSH concentrations, which may remain elevated until 2 to 4 years of age. One longitudinal study involving healthy full-term infant girls demonstrated 2 gonadotropin peaks in early infancy with 1 peak occurring around days 15 to 27 and a later peak occurring at days 164 to 165.[14]

As noted earlier, the human HPG axis manifests an on-off-on pattern (**Fig. 2**). The biological basis and rationale for transient post-natal HPG axis activity during the first few months of life are enigmatic. At birth, the brain is still plastic with ongoing development. Most axon and synapse formations are completed during the first year of life. Does this transient HPG axis activity imprint areas in the brain to influence future patterns of gonadotropin secretion? Do neonatal gonadal hormones affect future fertility, gender identity, sexual orientation, behaviors, and risk for autism spectrum dysfunction? Data are accruing regarding patterns of hormone secretion during the first 6 months of life. Nevertheless, the factors that initiate and terminate this transient HPG axis activity and maintain the quiescence of the HPG axis until the onset of puberty remain indeterminate.

GONADARCHE AND GONADS
Ovaries

Ovaries are responsible for hormone secretion, oogenesis/follicular maturation, and ovulation. For women, reproductive capacity is determined during gestation when

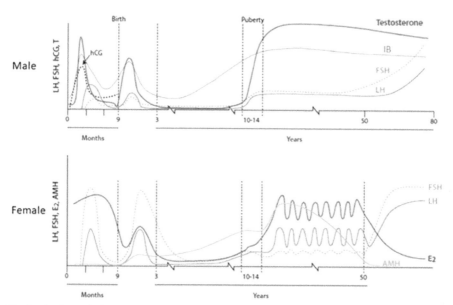

Fig. 2. The hypothalamic-pituitary-gonadal (HPG) axis during fetal and postnatal life. Circulating concentrations of gonadotropins, sex steroids, and inhibin B during the prenatal, immediate neonatal, prepubertal, pubertal, and adult time periods in boys and men (top panel). Gonadotropins, estradiol, and anti-Müllerian hormone during the same time period in girls and women (lower panel). AMH, anti-Müllerian hormone; E_2, estradiol; FSH, follicle-stimulating hormone; hCG, human chorionic gonadotropin; LH, luteinizing hormone; T, testosterone. (Reprinted with permission: Howard SR. Interpretation of reproductive hormones before, during and after the pubertal transition-Identifying health and disordered puberty. Clin Endocrinol (Oxf). 2021;95:702-15. https://doi.org/10.1111/cen.14578. PMID: 34368982.)

primordial follicles develop. Primordial follicles contain a small primary oocyte within a single layer of squamous granulosa cells. At birth, approximately 500,000 to 1 million primordial follicles are present. During the prepubertal years, primordial and preantral follicles predominate. Nevertheless, small gonadotropin-independent antral follicles can develop.

As would be anticipated, prepubertal ovaries are smaller than pubertal ovaries. Prepubertal ovaries show increased density of primordial follicles, less well-defined corticomedullary junction, and less commonly identified tunica albuginea compared to pubertal ovaries.[15] The prepubertal ovary contains a population of aberrant oocytes within primordial follicles. These oocytes are apparently eliminated prior to gonadarche because they are absent from the pubertal ovary. Factors governing the initial progression from primordial to primary follicles in the peri-pubertal ovary are poorly defined. Available data suggest that FSH and other factors influence oocyte chromatin and epigenetic factors such as histone methylation to advance oocyte development.[16]

Upon gonadarche, ovarian volume increases achieving maximum volume between menarche and age 16 years. FSH is essential to promote granulosa cell aromatase expression for the transition from primary to preantral follicles and estrogen synthesis. Among regularly cycling 16-year-old non-obese Danish girls, transabdominal ultrasound revealed the median ovarian volume to be 6.78 cm^3 with a median of 10 follicles (2.0–7.9 mm) per ovary.[17] Polycystic ovary morphology may be detected in healthy adolescent girls and is generally not associated with decreased ovulatory rate, hyperandrogenism, or metabolic abnormalities in this age group.

Testes

Sertoli cells, the first somatic cell type to differentiate in the embryonic testis, coordinate the differentiation of other testicular cells such as germ cells and Leydig cells. During embryonic testis development, fetal Sertoli cells aggregate surrounding the primordial germ cells, gonocytes, to form the testicular cords which will eventually develop into the seminiferous tubules in the adult testis. Throughout gestation and the neonatal period, Sertoli cells proliferate until terminal differentiation to adult Sertoli cells occurs at gonadarche.

By midgestation, most germ cells undergo transition to prespermatogonia. Spermatocytes, spermatids, and spermatozoa are absent from testes both during minipuberty and the prepubertal years. Despite circulating testosterone concentrations in the pubertal range during minipuberty, spermatogenesis fails to occur because Sertoli cells lack expression of the androgen receptor. Upon gonadarche with increased gonadotropin secretion, exponential increases in spermatogonia and testicular volume are apparent.

Two distinct populations of Leydig cells exist in mammals. Following birth, the fetal Leydig cells involute. With the onset of gonadarche, adult Leydig cells apparently derived from distinct stem cell progenitor cells arise.[18] Additional details regarding testicular development can be found elsewhere.[19]

FEEDBACK AT THE HYPOTHALAMUS AND PITUITARY
Sex Steroids

In males, LH promotes testicular testosterone synthesis and secretion. Testosterone circulates predominantly bound to sex hormone–binding globulin. Testosterone binds directly to the cytosolic androgen receptor. In some target tissues, such as the male genital skin and the prostate, testosterone is converted by the enzyme 5-alpha reductase to the more potent androgen, dihydrotesterone. Testosterone can also be converted to estradiol by the aromatase enzyme. Testosterone enables negative feedback inhibition of LH secretion by suppression of GnRH secretion via hypothalamic kisspeptin neurons and direct action on pituitary gonadotropes. Gonadotropin concentrations are typically not elevated in patients with complete androgen insensitivity. Measuring gonadotropins and testosterone during early infancy can help diagnose CHH in boys who present with micropenis.[20]

In females, LH promotes theca cell androstenedione synthesis followed by androstenedione diffusion to granulosa cells where FSH-stimulated aromatase converts it to estrogens. In females, sex steroid feedback affecting GnRH pulse frequency is essential to the menstrual cycle and involves both negative and positive feedback actions of ovarian steroids at both the hypothalamic and pituitary levels.

Gonadal Peptide Hormones

Anti-Mullerian hormone (AMH) is a homodimeric disulphide-linked glycoprotein member of the transforming growth factor-β family. Sertoli cells of the developing male fetus secrete AMH to promote in utero regression of the Mullerian ducts. With the onset of gonadarche, rising testosterone concentrations suppress Sertoli cell AMH production. In contrast, AMH concentrations are low in the developing female fetus. In the adolescent and adult woman, AMH is secreted by primary follicles and appears to negatively regulate the recruitment of resting follicles into active follicles. Thus, AMH limits the number of follicles maturing at any specific time point. Low AMH concentrations in girls with Turner syndrome or primary ovarian insufficiency suggest low follicular reserve.[21] High AMH concentrations in adolescent girls with irregular menses and hyperandrogenism suggest polycystic ovary syndrome.[22] Variable AMH assays and inconsistent AMH concentrations impede its usefulness in girls who are cancer survivors.[23]

Inhibin B, a member of the transforming growth factor-β family, is secreted by Sertoli cells in males and granulosa cells in females. Inhibin B is a glycoprotein heterodimer consisting of an inhibin alpha-subunit and an inhibin beta-B subunit. Inhibin B downregulates pituitary FSH synthesis. Inhibin B increases during minipuberty, remains low during childhood, and increases with gonadarche. In adult males, inhibin B reflects Sertoli cell mass and spermatogenic capacity.

Insulinlike peptide 3 (INSL3) is secreted by Leydig cells. During fetal life, INSL3 plays an important role in abdominal testicular descent. INSL3 secretion follows a similar pattern to LH with elevation during minipuberty, low concentrations during childhood, and rising again at gonadarche.

Gonadal peptide hormones can provide information regarding gonadal function. Low AMH and inhibin B concentrations in phenotypic boys are consistent with congenital anorchia or CHH. Inhibin B tends to be higher among boys with constitutional delay compared to those with CHH. Nevertheless, overlap between these groups occurs. The overlap in INSL3 concentrations limits its value in distinguishing individuals with CHH.

GENETICS OF PUBERTY

As noted earlier, the timing of puberty is heritable, with epidemiologic data indicating that genetic regulation accounts for 50% to 80% of the variation at age of pubertal onset. Age at puberty is associated with risk regarding long-term health outcomes such as breast cancer, cardiovascular disease, and osteopenia/osteoporosis. Large genome-wide association studies have identified genes that are associated with age at menarche in girls and age at voice break in boys. Over 1000 independent genetic signals associated with age at menarche were identified in multi-ancestry genetic analyses in approximately 800,000 women. These analyses implicated 660 genes in pubertal timing.[24]

SECULAR TRENDS TOWARD EARLIER PUBERTY

Over the past few decades, observations have suggested that puberty is starting at younger ages. Clinical studies examining ages at the onset of puberty depend on the criteria used to indicate puberty. For girls, age at the onset of breast development and age at menarche are conventional markers of puberty in girls. For boys, age at voice change has been used as a marker.[25]

Several longitudinal studies including the Breast Cancer and the Environment Research Program have noted a decrease in the age at the onset of breast development and a smaller decrease in the age at menarche.[26,27] The onset of breast development was assessed both through observation and palpation; however, gonadotropin concentrations were not included in these studies. Most of these studies have suggested that thelarche now occurs earlier than in the 1960s;[28] however, the age of menarche has remained relatively stable over recent decades, resulting in a longer interval between thelarche and menarche.[29] Several factors have been implicated as potential contributors to this earlier onset of puberty including obesity both in boys and girls,[30,31] environmental factors,[32] stress and perinatal growth,[33] and epigenetic factors. Internationally adopted girls seem to be at a higher risk of developing precocious puberty.[34] Environmental factors include exposure to substances which may mimic and/or antagonize endogenous sex steroid action, synthesis, or degradation, termed endocrine-disrupting chemicals (EDCs), many of which (like phthalates and phenols) are found in common household products.[32] Exposure to EDCs may occur by direct absorption through the skin, inhalation, or ingestion, and the effects can be cumulative due to consistent or repeated use of these products as well as potential joint effects of exposure to multiple chemicals across different chemical classes.

SUMMARY

Our understanding of the physiology of pubertal development, both in males and females has expanded over the past decades. Genetic, environmental, nutritional, and metabolic factors can influence the onset and tempo of puberty. Important findings include augmented knowledge of HPG axis function, discovery of the kisspeptin system, and the role of KNDy neurons in regulating hypothalamic GnRH secretion.

CLINICS CARE POINTS

- Genetic, metabolic, nutritional, environmental, ethnic, geographic, and economic factors influence the onset and tempo of pubertal development.
- The expansion of knowledge regarding how the timing and tempo of puberty relate to adult health status is important and should be further explored.
- An improved understanding of gametogenesis will enable successful fertility preservation for prepubertal children affected with disorders that would impact future fertility.

DISCLOSURE

The authors have nothing to disclose.

REFERENCES

1. Abreu AP, Kaiser UB. Pubertal development and regulation. Lancet Diabetes Endocrinol 2016;4(3):254–64.
2. Fuqua JS, Eugster EA. History of Puberty: Normal and Precocious. Horm Res Paediatr 2022;95(6):568–78.
3. Plant TM. Recognition that sustained pituitary gonadotropin secretion requires pulsatile GnRH stimulation: a Pittsburgh Saga. F S Rep 2023;4(2 Suppl):3–7.
4. Faienza MF, Urbano F, Moscogiuri LA, et al. Genetic, epigenetic and enviromental influencing factors on the regulation of precocious and delayed puberty. Front Endocrinol 2022;13:1019468.
5. Uenoyama Y, Tsukamura H. KNDy neurones and GnRH/LH pulse generation: Current understanding and future aspects. J Neuroendocrinol 2023;35(9):e13285.
6. Rege J, Turcu AF, Kasa-Vubu JZ, et al. 11-Ketotestosterone Is the Dominant Circulating Bioactive Androgen During Normal and Premature Adrenarche. J Clin Endocrinol Metab 2018;103(12):4589–98.
7. Breslow E, Taylor A, Chan CL, et al. 11-Oxygenated Androgen Metabolite Concentrations Are Affected by Pubertal Progression and Obesity. Horm Res Paediatr 2023;96(4):412–22.

8. Remer T, Boye KR, Hartmann MF, et al. Urinary markers of adrenarche: reference values in healthy subjects, aged 3-18 years. J Clin Endocrinol Metab 2005;90(4): 2015–21.

9. Marshall WA, Tanner JM. Variations in the pattern of pubertal changes in boys. Arch Dis Child 1970;45(239):13–23.

10. Marshall WA, Tanner JM. Variations in pattern of pubertal changes in girls. Arch Dis Child 1969;44(235):291–303.

11. Busch AS, Hollis B, Day FR, et al. Voice break in boys-temporal relations with other pubertal milestones and likely causal effects of BMI. Hum Reprod 2019; 34(8):1514–22.

12. Duittoz AH, Forni PE, Giacobini P, et al. Development of the gonadotropin-releasing hormone system. J Neuroendocrinol 2022;34(5):e13087.

13. Forest MG, Sizonenko PC, Cathiard AM, et al. Hypophyso-gonadal function in humans during the first year of life. 1. Evidence for testicular activity in early infancy. J Clin Invest 1974;53(3):819–28.

14. Ljubicic ML, Busch AS, Upners EN, et al. A Biphasic Pattern of Reproductive Hormones in Healthy Female Infants: The COPENHAGEN Minipuberty Study. J Clin Endocrinol Metab 2022;107(9):2598–605.

15. Tsui EL, Harris CJ, Rowell EE, et al. Human ovarian gross morphology and sub-anatomy across puberty: insights from tissue donated during fertility preservation. F S Rep 2023;4(2):196–205.

16. Wasserzug Pash P, Karavani G, Reich E, et al. Pre-pubertal oocytes harbor altered histone modifications and chromatin configuration. Front Cell Dev Biol 2022;10:1060440.

17. Assens M, Dyre L, Henriksen LS, et al. Menstrual Pattern, Reproductive Hormones, and Transabdominal 3D Ultrasound in 317 Adolescent Girls. J Clin Endocrinol Metab 2020;105(9).

18. Kilcoyne KR, Smith LB, Atanassova N, et al. Fetal programming of adult Leydig cell function by androgenic effects on stem/progenitor cells. Proc Natl Acad Sci U S A 2014;111(18):E1924–32.

19. Makela JA, Koskenniemi JJ, Virtanen HE, et al. Testis Development. Endocr Rev 2019;40(4):857–905.

20. Swee DS, Quinton R. Congenital Hypogonadotrophic Hypogonadism: Minipuberty and the Case for Neonatal Diagnosis. Front Endocrinol 2019;10:97.

21. Lunding SA, Aksglaede L, Anderson RA, et al. AMH as Predictor of Premature Ovarian Insufficiency: A Longitudinal Study of 120 Turner Syndrome Patients. J Clin Endocr Metab 2015;100(7):E1030–8.

22. Rudnicka E, Kunicki M, Calik-Ksepka A, et al. Anti-Mullerian Hormone in Pathogenesis, Diagnostic and Treatment of PCOS. Int J Mol Sci 2021;22(22).

23. Torella M, Riemma G, De Franciscis P, et al. Serum Anti-Mullerian Hormone Levels and Risk of Premature Ovarian Insufficiency in Female Childhood Cancer Survivors: Systematic Review and Network Meta-Analysis. Cancers 2021;13(24).

24. Kentistou KA, Kaisinger LR, Stankovic S, et al. Understanding the genetic complexity of puberty timing across the allele frequency spectrum. medRxiv 2023. https://doi.org/10.1101/2023.06.14.23291322.

25. Brix N, Ernst A, Lauridsen LLB, et al. Timing of puberty in boys and girls: A population-based study. Paediatr Perinat Epidemiol 2019;33(1):70–8.

26. Biro FM, Greenspan LC, Galvez MP, et al. Onset of breast development in a longitudinal cohort. Pediatrics 2013;132(6):1019–27.

27. Biro FM, Pajak A, Wolff MS, et al. Age of Menarche in a Longitudinal US Cohort. J Pediatr Adolesc Gynecol 2018;31(4):339–45.

28. Eckert-Lind C, Busch AS, Petersen JH, et al. Worldwide Secular Trends in Age at Pubertal Onset Assessed by Breast Development Among Girls: A Systematic Review and Meta-analysis. JAMA Pediatr 2020;174(4):e195881.

29. Sorensen K, Mouritsen A, Aksglaede L, et al. Recent secular Trends in Pubertal Timing: Implications for Evaluation and Diagnosis of Precocious Puberty. Horm Res Paediatr 2012;77:137–45.

30. Brix N, Ernst A, Lauridsen LLB, et al. Childhood overweight and obesity and timing of puberty in boys and girls: cohort and sibling-matched analyses. Int J Epidemiol 2020;49(3):834–44.

31. Kaplowitz PB. Link between body fat and the timing of puberty. Pediatrics 2008; 121(Suppl 3):S208–17.

32. Taylor KW, Howdeshell KL, Bommarito PA, et al. Systematic evidence mapping informs a class-based approach to assessing personal care products and pubertal timing. Environ Int 2023;181:108307.

33. Persson I, Ahlsson F, Ewald U, et al. Influence of perinatal factors on the onset of puberty in boys and girls: implications for interpretation of link with risk of long term diseases. Am J Epidemiol 1999;150(7):747–55.

34. Teilmann G, Petersen JH, Gormsen M, et al. Early puberty in internationally adopted girls: hormonal and clinical markers of puberty in 276 girls examined biannually over two years. Horm Res 2009;72(4):236–46.

Females with Breast Development before Three Years of Age

Paul B. Kaplowitz, MD, PhD[a], Peter A. Lee, MD, PhD[b],*

KEYWORDS

- Premature thelarche • Central precocious puberty • Breast development

KEY POINTS

- A very young girl with early breast development almost always has premature thelarche (PT) which may regress before 2 to 3 years with rare persistence beyond that age.
- PT may persist from birth or develop in the first few months of life as a consequence of estrogen secretion, which is sporadic, possibly as a consequence of "minipuberty."
- Only when changes progress markedly or when growth rate is clearly above normal range, should any testing be done to rule out central precocious puberty (CPP) or peripheral precocious puberty.
- Laboratory testing is not helpful except in the situation noted earlier because basal and gonadotropin-releasing hormone (GnRH)/GnRH analogue–stimulated luteinizing hormone levels can overlap with those seen in older children with CPP.
- Individual cases may occasionally be so complicated that the application of any guidelines may be problematic, but for most cases, the monitor-before-testing strategy works well.

INTRODUCTION

Premature thelarche (PT) is one of the most common benign variations of early pubertal development in girls. Primary care providers are often quite concerned about what may appear to be the onset of true puberty in a very young girl and order unnecessary testing which may further worry already-anxious parents. While pediatric endocrinologists are generally familiar with its presentation and benign course, there is still a tendency among some to order tests "just to make sure we're not missing something." Such testing may lead to further testing, such as gonadotropin-releasing hormone (GnRH)/ GnRH analogue (GnRHa) stimulation testing, in which responses are greater than during childhood and sometimes lead to inappropriate treatment.

[a] Division of Endocrinology, Children's National Hospital, George Washington School of Medicine and Health Sciences, 111 Michigan Avenue Northwest, Washington, DC 20010, USA;
[b] Division of Pediatric Endocrinology, Penn State School of Medicine, Milton S. Hershey Medical Center, 500 University Avenue, Hershey, PA 17033, USA
* Corresponding author. Penn State Health, 12 Briarcrest Square, Hershey, PA 17033.
E-mail address: plee@pennstatehealth.psu.edu

Endocrinol Metab Clin N Am 53 (2024) 195–201
https://doi.org/10.1016/j.ecl.2024.01.002
0889-8529/24/© 2024 Elsevier Inc. All rights reserved.
endo.theclinics.com

One coauthor has recently written a commentary including presenting the case for waiting before testing[1]; this article provides a more complete review of pertinent data, including recent publications. It is further worthy of note that a pediatric endocrinology fact sheet guideline for families (copyrighted in 2018 by the American Academy of Pediatrics and Pediatric Endocrine Society) regarding PT states that nonprogressive breast development noted in girls before 3 years of age should be observed, noting that menarche occurs at a normal age. The information provided herein is from multiple diverse studies of different study populations, some of which appear to be nonrepresentative. Hence, the reader is advised not to draw firm conclusions from any single study, but note that the authors have attempted to interpret the overall data. In this article, the authors highlight what is known and unknown about PT, areas of current debate (such as how often PT progresses to CPP), and why hormone testing and imaging should in most cases be avoided when there are no red flags.

DEFINITION AND CLINICAL PRESENTATION

PT is generally defined as breast development in a girl who is less than 8 years of age which does not progress during follow-up to central precocious puberty (CPP). Early reports indicate than it overall occurs in 20.0 per 100,000 girls, with 60% to 85% of the cases occurring by age 2 years.[2–4] Regression occurs in most over a period of 0.5 to 6 years, although regression was reported to be less common among girls with onset after 2 years.[2,5] Because the majority of girls who meet this definition are 3 year old or younger and are less likely to progress than the older girls, we will focus on this younger age group.

It is pertinent to remember that all newborns have breast buds. Mean diameters range from 4 to 18 mm (97%ile) and are larger in females than males.[6] The incidence of PT among 18-month-old girls in a cohort of 3140 girls in Sweden was 0.16%, and an evaluation from this age to 36 months found no progression although 2 were excluded from the study because of suspected CPP. A subset of only 24 with perhaps minimal progression was followed clinically and with estradiol levels. Among those, 4 were considered to have a cyclic course of progression and regression and were followed longer without any clear progression.[7] Clinical verification of PT[8] included the absence of a clear increase in breast size from Tanner stage 2 to 3 over a period of observation, verified by parents usually reporting little or no change since they first noticed breast tissue. In 1 study, the mean age at thelarche was 7.4 months, and the mean age at the first endocrine consultation was 19 months.[8] Thus, on average, nearly a year had passed between thelarche and the first endocrine visit, and in nearly all cases, breast development remained at stage 2.

Another helpful clue is that linear growth remains close to its previous percentile channel, demonstrating a lack of the growth acceleration expected in girls with CPP. The physical examination is normal except for a 1 to 2 cm bud of glandular breast tissue, although some girls with PT have more advanced breast development. No vaginal discharge and red (non-estrogenized) rather than pink (estrogenized) vaginal mucosa are noted. It is pertinent to measure diameters of the nipple and areolae as a baseline since persistent estrogen stimulation will increase the diameter of both.[4,9,10] During follow-up, breast development can either regress (up to 60%) or remain unchanged.

ETIOLOGY

The etiology of PT remains poorly understood. One theory is that the ovaries of girls with PT contain small follicles which can produce small amounts of estradiol prior to regressing, but this is found only in some PT girls.[11] However, it is likely that estrogen secretion is episodic.

It is also possible that the persistence or appearance of PT is a manifestation of the poorly understood phenomenon of increased hypothalamic-pituitary-ovarian (HPO) activity called "minipuberty"[12] in girls, when gonadotropins rise and estradiol undergoes cyclic fluctuations in the first 3 to 6 months of life.[13] Girls with PT from as young as 0.4 years have inhibin B and follicle-stimulating hormone (FSH) concentrations higher than age-matched controls and positively correlated with each other.[11] This is evidence that there is enhanced follicular development in PT. While some estrogenic stimulation of breast tissue is common in the neonatal period, it is unclear why this would regress in most girls but persist in girls with PT.

CURRENT EVIDENCE
How Often Does Typical Premature Thelarche Progress to Central Precocious Puberty?

This is an area of controversy, as published reports vary widely in the frequency of progression, but the criteria used to define progression differ from study to study. For example, 1 report from 2012 suggested that 20 out of 67 girls (29.1%) with PT aged less than 2 years progressed to early puberty, which was defined as when Tanner breast stage had advanced in the course of the 1 year follow-up or if the absolute growth velocity standard deviation score (SDS) was greater than 1 SDS. However, these patients did not have hormonal confirmation of CPP.[14] The largest and best study of this issue was that of Bizzarri,[15] which started with a group of 450 girls, 302 of whom had appearance of breast development in the first 6 months of life and 51 between 6 and 12 months; nearly all of these girls had complete or partial regression during follow-up done every 3 months, and none progressed to CPP. Another 97 girls had either onset after 12 months of age or 1 sign suggestive of progression and underwent complete hormonal and imaging evaluation. In the end, 9 of these 97 with progression were diagnosed with CPP (3 had hypothalamic hamartomas) and another 3 were diagnosed with peripheral precocious puberty. Thus, for the entire group of 450 girls with early onset of breast development before age 3, 9 (2%) progressed to CPP, a much lower figure than most studies. The authors' own experience from their clinical practices, covering over 1000 patients over a period of 35 and 50 years, is that no girl initially labeled as PT was later diagnosed with CPP. Thus, while the exact rate of progression is uncertain, the authors would argue that progression from PT to CPP is rare.

How Helpful Are Basal and Stimulated Gonadotropin Levels, Bone Age, and Pelvic Ultrasound in Distinguishing Premature Thelarche from Central Precocious Puberty?

Gonadotropin-releasing hormone or gonadotrophin-releasing hormone analogue stimulation testing
The differentiation of PT from CPP among children after infancy involves onset and progression of pubertal physical changes, accelerated growth rate, and, depending on duration, advanced skeletal age. The standard for verifying CPP is gonadotropin responses to GnRH stimulation testing, especially the LH rise.[16] However, stimulation testing during infancy has not been well studied and available data have not been useful in differentiating PT from CPP. The following summaries of studies suggest that GnRH or GnRHa stimulation testing and skeletal ages are not useful and such testing should be avoided unless rapidly progressive puberty and accelerated growth rates are occurring.

Published data regarding the diagnosis of CPP during infancy are lacking. Data, some previously unpublished, are included here primarily to illustrate that such testing is not indicated among patients presenting with clinical evidence of only PT. These data also illustrate that such testing generally shows levels within the overlapping prepubertal and pubertal response range, with dramatic exceptions among some with hypothalamic hamartomas.

Reports of GnRH/GnRHa testing during the first 2 or 3 years of life among those with PT:

1. An early study[17] used the most sensitive assay at the time (dissociation-enhanced lanthanide fluorescence immunoassay [DELFIA]) with LH and FSH before and after GnRH stimulation. Results with this assay were considerably higher than with current sensitive assays. Nevertheless, the levels compared with older children having CPP were considerably higher and demonstrated a more active HPO axis.
   a. Peak LH levels after GnRH among infants with CPP ranged from 35.3 to 81.7 IU/L (including patients with hypothalamic hamartomas); among those without CPP, the peak levels ranged from 3.3 to 13.1 IU/L. Among 9 females older than 3 years (mean 6.7) with CPP, stimulated LH ranged from 15.0 to 47.9 IU/L. Baseline levels of LH overlapped.
   b. Baseline and stimulated FSH responses overlapped for the infants with CPP and PT.
   c. Baseline estradiol levels were undetectable ($\leq$5 pg/mL) among all non-CPP and ranged from greater than 5 to 90 pg/mL (median 20) among those with CPP.
   d. Growth rates (except among those with hamartomas) and skeletal age SDS were not helpful and sometimes misleading.
      Two of the first patients evaluated were started on GnRHa therapy based on skeletal age advancement, but treatment was discontinued at age 2 years and they were followed for 3 more years without any evidence of CPP.
      Review of clinical findings among these infants indicates those with CPP, both with and without hypothalamic hamartomas, presented with dramatic robust physical progression of puberty. Screening testing for those with PT is likely to be misleading and can lead to subsequent expensive evaluation.
2. Bizzarri[15] found CPP among 9 of 97 girls less than 3 years of age with prolonged follow-up and complete hormone testing; of the 97, 85 were verified to have PT, 9 with CPP, and 3 with peripheral precocious puberty. Peak responses to GnRH testing in girls with PT were a median of 3.81 IU/L (range 0.1–22.6) and for girls with CPP, a median of 24.48 IU/L (range 7.7–144). The response for only 1 of the 85 who had PT overlapped the CPP range, and also only 1 of the 9 with CPP overlapped the PT range. Thus, the results illustrate the limited value of GnRH/GnRHa testing.
3. An abstract presented in 2013[18] reported GnRH stimulation testing among 12 infants, 6 of whom were diagnosed with CPP. However, 4 of the 6 with CPP had hypothalamic hamartomas.
4. A report[4] of 191 girls with PT, including 9 greater than 3 years of age included body mass index SDS, basal and GnRH-stimulated FSH and LH, and sex-hormone binding globulin. The authors report that all of these parameters were useful in differentiating precocious puberty from PT. They also found 4 who were less than 2 year old who had CPP, which is an unexpected number, especially since none were found to have hypothalamic hamartomas. However, there was overlap of both basal and peak stimulated LH values between infants not diagnosed with CPP as well as

older children with and without PT, in addition to the expected overlap of FSH. Nevertheless, these authors conclude that PT "is most often a physiologic condition that stabilizes or regresses spontaneously."

5. A Turkish report (**Fig. 1, Table 1**) from 2020 studying 30 PT patients less than 3.0 years old[19] noted that baseline and peak LH values among 30 girls with PT less than 3 years were similar to pubertal values. Ten of the 30 PT patients had basal LH levels greater than 0.3 IU/L. The peak LH/FSH ratio was more useful, with a mean of 0.17 ± 0.09 with all ≤ 0.43. Thus, the LH/FSH ratio was much more accurate in confirming a diagnosis of PT than the peak LH ≥ 5 IU/L. Therefore, if testing is done, which the authors feel is rarely necessary, the peak LH/FSH ratio should be evaluated.

How Helpful Are Bone Age and Pelvic Ultrasound Studies?

Three studies[16,17,19] all showed that bone age advancement could not reliably distinguish between PT and CPP. While there are fewer studies of pelvic ultrasound, 1 study did find that the mean longitudinal diameter of the uterus was greater in the 9 girls with CPP than the 85 extensively evaluated girls with PT, though there was much overlap.[15]

SUGGESTED CLINICAL APPROACH AND COUNSELING

A very important consideration in managing typical cases of PT is how to communicate with the parents and the referring provider. One should make clear that PT is not an uncommon finding in girls 3 years and younger and that it is rare that early breast development will progress rapidly and require further evaluation. Hormonal and imaging studies are, therefore, generally not needed at the time of the first visit, and parents may be told that in nearly all cases, menarche will occur at a time within the typical age of menarche.

There are 2 ways to manage follow-up monitoring. The child can be seen in 4 to 6 months by the endocrine provider who can assess the growth rate and check on the amount of breast tissue. It is helpful if the diameter of the breast tissue has been measured at the first visit for comparison. If there has been no change, further follow-up can be passed on to the referring provider. The parents and the provider should be informed that if the child experiences rapid growth, particularly if the amount of breast tissue seems to be increasing, then prompt referral back to the endocrine provider is needed. If the endocrine provider has a low level of concern, another option

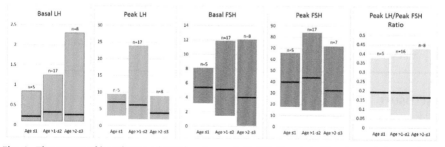

Fig. 1. The range of basal LH and FSH levels, peak GnRH-stimulated levels, and the peak LH/peak FSH ratios[19] together with the crossline in each bar indicating the median (basal and peak LH) and mean (basal and peak FSH, LH/FSH ratio) levels. Note that the scales are different for each plot. FSH, follicle-stimulating hormone; GnRH, gonadotropin hormone-releasing hormone; LH, luteinizing hormone.

Table 1
Summary of data from girls with premature thelarche less than 3 years of age

Number of Girls	30
Age (y)	1.3[a] (0.8–3.0)
Bone Age (y)	1.4[a] (1.0–2.0)
BA − CA (y)	0.3[a] (0.1–1.3)
Breast stage II or III	8 stage II & 22 stage III
Height SDS	1.5 (0.5–3.0)
Height velocity SDS	−0.19 (−2.1–3.7)
Basal LH	n = 15 < 0.3 & n = 15 > 0.3 IU/L
Peak LH	n = 12 < 5 IU/L & n = 18 > 5 IU/L
Peak LH/Peak FSH ratio	Range 0.05–0.43

Abbreviations: BA, bone age; CA, chronological age; FSH, follicle-stimulating hormone; LH, luteinizing hormone; SDS, standard deviation score.
[a] Median ± Range.
Adapted from Seymen Karabulut G, Atar M, Çizmecioğlu Jones FM, Hatun Ş. Girls with Premature Thelarche Younger than 3 Years of Age May Have Stimulated Luteinizing Hormone Greater than 10 IU/L. J Clin Res Pediatr Endocrinol. 2020 Nov 25;12(4):377-382. https://doi.org/10.4274/jcrpe.galenos.2020.2019.0202. Epub 2020 Apr 29. PMID: 32349465; PMCID: PMC7711634.

is to turn over follow-up to the referring provider after the first visit. While it is true that rare cases of CPP present at a very young age, particularly those due to a hypothalamic hamartoma, most cases will present with red flags that will prompt early testing and diagnosis.

CLINICS CARE POINTS

- Early breast development (PT) is most common during the first 2 to 3 years of life and almost always is a self-limiting condition.
  - Almost always, only observation for progression and growth rate is required.
  - Data regarding basal and peak GnRHa-stimulated LH and FSH levels and FSH/LH ratios verify that such testing is only indicated when breast development progresses rapidly or growth rate is clearly excessive.
  - Skeletal age x-rays are seldom helpful.
- Children older than 3 years presenting with breast development should be observed to determine whether changes progress and other physical evidence of puberty is present.
  - This allows determination of whether the normal variant of PT is present or if clear progression indicates that central and peripheral precocious puberty need to be excluded.
  - Assessment of central and peripheral precocious puberty are presented in other articles in this volume.

DISCLOSURE

The authors have nothing to disclose.

REFERENCES

1. Kaplowitz PB. For premature thelarche and premature adrenarche, the case for waiting before testing. Horm Res Paediatr 2020;93(9–10):573–6. Epub 2020 Dec 22. PMID: 33352558.

2. Van Winter JT, Noller KL, Zimmerman D, et al. Natural history of premature the-larche in Olmsted County, Minnesota, 1940 to 1984. J Pediatr 1990 Feb;116(2): 278–80.
3. Ilicki A, Prager Lewin R, Kauli R, et al. Premature thelarche–natural history and sex hormone secretion in 68 girls. Acta Paediatr Scand 1984 Nov;73(6):756–62.
4. Volta C, Bernasconi S, Cisternino M, et al. Isolated premature thelarche and the-larche variant: clinical and auxological follow-up of 119 girls. J Endocrinol Invest 1998 Mar;21(3):180–3.
5. Verrotti A, Ferrari M, Morgese G, et al. Premature thelarche: a long-term follow-up. Gynecol Endocrinol 1996 Aug;10(4):241–7.
6. Shah R, Alshaikh B, Schall JI, et al. Endocrine-sensitive physical endpoints in newborns: ranges and predictors. Pediatr Res 2021 Feb;89(3):660–6.
7. Österbrand M, Fors H, Norjavaara E. Prevalence of premature thelarche at 18 months of age: a population- and hospital-based study of prevalence and inci-dence in girls born at northern älvsborg county hospital in Sweden. Horm Res Paediatr 2019;91(3):203–9.
8. Kaplowitz PB, Mehra R. Clinical characteristics of children referred for signs of early puberty before age 3. J Pediatr Endocrinol Metab 2015 Sep;28(9–10): 1139–44.
9. Rohn RD. Nipple (papilla) development in puberty: longitudinal observations in girls. Pediatrics 1987 May;79(5):745–7.
10. Stanhope R, Abdulwahid NA, Adams J, et al. Studies of gonadotrophin pulsatility and pelvic ultrasound examinations distinguish between isolated premature the-larche and central precocious puberty. Eur J Pediatr 1986 Aug;145(3):190–4.
11. Crofton PM, Evans NE, Wardhaugh B, et al. Evidence for increased ovarian follic-ular activity in girls with premature thelarche. Clin Endocrinol 2005 Feb;62(2): 205–9.
12. Becker M, Hesse V. Minipuberty: Why Does it Happen? Horm Res Paediatr 2020; 93(2):76–84.
13. Lanciotti L, Cofini M, Leonardi A, et al. Up-To-Date Review About Minipuberty and Overview on Hypothalamic-Pituitary-Gonadal Axis Activation in Fetal and Neonatal Life. Front Endocrinol 2018 Jul 23;9:410.
14. Uçar A, Saka N, Baş F, et al. Is premature thelarche in the first two years of life transient? J Clin Res Pediatr Endocrinol 2012 Sep;4(3):140–5.
15. Bizzarri C, Spadoni GL, Bottaro G, et al. The response to gonadotropin releasing hormone (GnRH) stimulation test does not predict the progression to true preco-cious puberty in girls with onset of premature thelarche in the first three years of life. J Clin Endocrinol Metab 2014 Feb;99(2):433–9.
16. Pescovitz OH, Hench KD, Barnes KM, et al. Premature thelarche and central pre-cocious puberty: the relationship between clinical presentation and the gonado-tropin response to luteinizing hormone-releasing hormone. J Clin Endocrinol Metab 1988 Sep;67(3):474–9.
17. Gschwend S, Lee PA. Precocious puberty during infancy: Diagnosis and GnRHa treatment. 3rd International Symposium on GnRH analogues. Gynecol Endocrinol 1993;7(Suppl 3):73.
18. Wang Y, Liang L, Fang Y, et al. Poster Presentation-A clinical follow-up study of premature thelarche in infants under the age of two. Int'l J Pediatr Endocrinol 2013;2013(Suppl 1):P129. http://www.ijpeonline.com/content/2013/S1/P129.
19. Seymen Karabulut G, Atar M, Çizmecioğlu Jones FM, et al. Girls with Premature Thelarche Younger than 3 Years of Age May Have Stimulated Luteinizing Hor-mone Greater than 10 IU/L. J Clin Res Pediatr Endocrinol 2020;12(4):377–82.

Premature Pubarche
A Pragmatic Approach

Paul B. Kaplowitz, MD, PhD*

KEYWORDS

- Premature pubarche • Premature adrenarche
- Nonclassical congenital adrenal hyperplasia • Pubic hair of infancy • Bone age

KEY POINTS

- Premature pubarche (PP) is a common and benign variant of early puberty most often seen in 5-year-old to 9-year-old children, characterized by pubic and/or axillary hair, axillary odor, and often tall stature and increased body mass index.
- Laboratory studies typically show a modest elevation of dehydroepiandrosterone sulfate with normal testosterone and 17-hydroxyprogesterone, except for the occasional case of mild nonclassic congenital adrenal hyperplasia.
- Bone age is often advanced, but rarely indicates serious pathology.
- It is suggested that for the typical cases of PP without red flags, laboratory testing and bone age X rays be withheld at the first visit, with follow-up either by the pediatric endocrine provider or the referring provider, to identify the rare case with a more serious diagnosis.

INTRODUCTION

Premature pubarche (PP) is a common benign variant in which there is early appearance of pubic and/or axillary hair, as well as other mild signs of androgen excess.[1] There are many studies looking at the natural history of PP and the low frequency of pathologic diagnoses in children with early appearance of pubic hair. However, there are significant differences in how providers approach this situation and how laboratory tests and bone age (BA) X rays are used to rule out other conditions which may present with early pubic hair. For example, Rosenfield,[2] in his 2021 review, while conceding that at least 90% of PP cases are due to premature adrenarche (PA), includes a long list of virilizing disorders to rule out, including many rare adrenal disorders, and recommends as a minimum workup a BA and the 3 most commonly ordered steroids discussed in the following sections. In this article, the author will discuss the typical clinical presentation of this problem and present evidence to support the position

Division of Endocrinology, Children's National Hospital, Washington, DC, USA
* Corresponding author.
E-mail address: pkaplowi@childrensnational.org

Endocrinol Metab Clin N Am 53 (2024) 203–209
https://doi.org/10.1016/j.ecl.2024.02.001
0889-8529/24/© 2024 Elsevier Inc. All rights reserved.

that, in most cases, no laboratory tests or X rays are needed to confirm a diagnosis of benign PP.

DEFINING PREMATURE PUBARCHE AND PREMATURE ADRENARCHE

The commonly accepted definition of PP is the appearance of pubic hair prior to age 8 in girls and prior to age 9 in boys; however, many studies have found this to be very common in the United States, especially in Black and Hispanic girls, due to their earlier development of pubertal milestones.[3] Over 90% of cases of PP are due to PA[2], which is due to an earlier-than-normal increase in secretion of adrenal androgens such as dehydroepiandrosterone and its sulfated form (DHEA-S), an event known as adrenarche, as discussed in (see Kanthi Bangalore Krishna and Selma F. Witchel's article, "Normal Puberty," in this issue). The appearance of pubic hair can occur either before, at the same time, or later than other signs of puberty (breast development in girls and penile and testicular enlargement in boys), so these findings represent 2 independent physiologic processes.

One condition which should not be confused with PP is generalized hypertrichosis, or a diffuse increase in body hair.[4] Such patients do not have hair limited to areas which are sex hormone dependent (beard area, axilla, lower abdomen, and genital area). On history, it is often found that a parent (typically the father) also has excess body hair.

CLINICAL PRESENTATION

The typical patient with PP is between the ages of 5 and 8 years and is referred because of concerns with pubic hair (usually Tanner stage 2 at the first visit) along the labia or scrotum and spreading over the pubic symphysis. In most studies, boys make up about 20% of patients with PP. The clitoris or penis is not enlarged. Pubic hair is often accompanied by the appearance of axillary hair and the characteristic adult-type axillary odor, which is frequently noted 6 to 12 months prior to pubic hair. Many patients are already using deodorants. Mild acne is occasionally seen. The growth chart will often show height above the 90th percentile, and in some cases, the growth rate will be above normal for age. Weight and body mass index (BMI) are often increased for age, and rapid weight gain is common. A slow increase over time in the amount of pubic hair is often seen between the time it was first noted and the time of the first endocrine consultation. The family history is often negative for others with an early appearance of pubic hair.

NATURAL HISTORY

During follow-up, there is typically a slow but steady increase in the amount of hair in the genital region with no other signs of androgen excess. Growth usually follows the patient's percentile channel, but more rapid growth (7–10 cm/year) may be seen and was documented in 17% of PP patients in 1 study.[5] The onset of puberty and age at menarche has been found to be similar to population means.[6] While advanced BA and tall stature were frequent during follow-up, adult height correlated with height prediction at diagnosis and was often above mid-parental height. However, when the same group divided PP patients according to birthweight, they found that the low birthweight subset had menarche an average of 8 to 10 months earlier and shorter adult stature than the higher birthweight group.[7]

Studies from Spain have shown that girls with PP may develop polycystic ovary syndrome with irregular periods and insulin resistance in their teen years, especially girls born with low birthweight[8]

LABORATORY FINDINGS

The tests most often ordered by pediatric endocrinologists to evaluate PP are DHEA-S, the storage form of DHEA; 17-hydroxyprogesterone (17-OHP); and testosterone. DHEA-S levels are generally elevated for age but appropriate for the stage of pubic hair and are usually in the range of 30 to 150 µg/dL. Levels in excess of 200 µg/dL should increase concern for a diagnosis other than PA. Testosterone is prepubertal (usually<10 ng/dL), and random 17-OHP, to screen for nonclassic congenital adrenal hyperplasia (NC-CAH) as discussed in the following sections, is normal. Providers often order luteinizing hormone and follicle-stimulating hormone to rule out central precocious puberty, but in the absence of breast development in girls or testicular enlargement in boys, those tests are unnecessary. The pros and cons of ordering these tests are summarized in **Table 1**. When a BA is ordered, it shows an advance of greater than 1 year in most and greater than 2 years in many and yet as previously mentioned, adult height is typically normal. The author discusses in the following sections whether a BA X ray should be done routinely.

BENIGN GENITAL HAIR OF INFANCY: A VARIANT OF PREMATURE PUBARCHE?

In 1989, the first cases of genital hair in infants (all boys) were reported, followed by another 5 cases in 1992 including both sexes.[9,10] What was unique about these children was that the hair was very fine and located along the labia in females and on the scrotum in boys, with no hair around the pubic symphysis and no other signs of androgen excess. No evidence of a serious underlying endocrinopathy was found. In 2006, a larger study reviewed 11 cases and concluded that while the etiology was unclear, the condition appeared to be benign.[11] In 2007, a series of 12 cases was reported (9 females/3 males) with panels of 9 steroids performed by liquid chromatography-tandem mass spectrometry. The only abnormality found was that 6 of 12 had levels of DHEA-S which were somewhat above the infant normal range (ie, >15 µg/dL).[12] During follow up, genital hair persisted for 6 months to 2 years in most and disappeared in 2. In a 2015 study of 275 infants at 1 urban hospital presenting with signs of puberty under age 3, 69 (56 girls and 13 boys) had genital hair in infancy. Again, many but not all had a mild elevation of DHEA-S.[13] This condition remains poorly understood, and it is unclear why its incidence has apparently increased since 1990. It is most likely a benign variant of PP occurring at a very early age, as more serious diagnoses have not been made during follow-up. Therefore, reassurance of the parents rather than extensive testing should be the cornerstone of management.

CONTROVERSIES ABOUT MISSED DIAGNOSES

NC-CAH, or late-onset congenital adrenal hyperplasia (CAH), due to a mild deficiency of the enzyme 21-hydroxylase is the most common alternative diagnosis made in children with PP, with 2 large studies finding that approximately 4% to 5% of such patients have hormonal evidence of NC-CAH based on adrenocorticotropic hormone (ACTH) testing.[14,15] In the study which found that 4% of 238 subjects with PP had NC-CAH, all those patients had random 17-OHP of at least 6 nmol/L (200 ng/dL), which the investigators argued made ACTH stimulation testing unnecessary in most cases.[14] A more recent study in which 6 of 111 patients with PP and a BA advanced by at least 1 year were diagnosed with NC-CAH, the investigators also concluded that a basal 17-OHP of greater than 200 ng/dL was a useful screening test.[16]

   It is controversial as to whether screening for NC-CAH should be performed in all children with PP due to concerns about missing a potentially treatable condition.

Test	Why to Order	Why Not to Order
Table 1 Common tests ordered for premature pubarche: pros and cons		
DHEA-S	An elevation confirms that PP is likely due to PA	The result is unlikely to change management.
17-OHP	A level > 200 ng/dL makes NC-CAH more likely and would prompt an ACTH stimulation test	Diagnosing NC-CAH is unlikely to be of benefit to a child without evidence of virilization other than pubic hair.
Testosterone	An elevated level raises concern for a virilizing disorder such as a gonadal tumor	It is rare for a child with PP but no other signs of virilization to have an elevated level.
LH and FSH	May help diagnose CPP	A child with pubic hair only and no breast development or enlarged testes does not have CPP.

Abbreviations: ACTH, adrenocorticotropic hormone; CPP, central precocious puberty; DHEA-S, dehydroepiandrosterone sulfate; FSH, follicle-stimulating hormone; LH, luteinizing hormone; NC-CAH, nonclassic congenital adrenal hyperplasia; PA, premature adrenarche; PP, premature pubarche; 17-OHP, 17-hydroxyprogesterone.

While some children with NC-CAH clearly have clinical and growth evidence of hyperandrogenism and may benefit from treatment with glucocorticoids, many do not. Their height may be similar to children with PA and normal ACTH testing, though they tend to present at a younger age, be thinner. and have a more advanced BA.[15] Not testing any children with PA would likely miss a few children with NC-CAH. However, there are currently no studies showing that children with NC-CAH who are clinically indistinguishable from those with normal 17-OHP levels benefit from treatment in terms of prevention of more severe manifestations of androgen excess and short adult stature. One recent European multicenter study looked retrospectively at a group of 192 NC-CAH patients, mostly treated with glucocorticoids, who achieved adult heights only modestly below the normal range. However, the smaller untreated group (11% of the total) achieved normal and slightly greater adult heights than the treated group ($P = .053$).[17] While it is likely that the untreated group had a milder presentation as they were significantly older at diagnosis, it is clear that withholding treatment of NC-CAH does not inevitably lead to rapidly advancing BA and short stature. The potential risk of treatment is that even modest doses of glucocorticoid replacement may slow growth and increase weight gain, at least in the short term, as illustrated in a case discussed in a recent commentary.[18] The author was consulted on an 8.5-year-old girl from an Ashkenazi Jewish family who had axillary odor starting at 7.5 years and pubic hair starting at 8 years. Height was 35th percentile, and BA was advanced 2 years. Her DHEA-S was 39, testosterone 13, and random 17- OHP 3500 ng/dL with an increase to 5590 ng/dL after ACTH stimulation testing. Genotyping revealed that the girl, her 7-year-old sister who also had pubic hair, and the mother all tested homozygous for a common mutation associated with NC-CAH (V281L), and the father was a carrier. The mother was 5'2", slightly below her target height of 5'4", and was obviously fertile. Their endocrine provider recommended treatment with hydrocortisone at a dose of 13 mg/m²/day, and at subsequent visits, their growth slowed and weight gain increased. Stopping hydrocortisone was suggested, following which linear growth improved and weight gain slowed. Thus, one cannot assume that treatment of NC-CAH has no risks. Also, the cost of follow-up visits and frequent monitoring of 17-OHP and other steroids can be substantial over time, making the argument for the benefits relative to the costs of early NC-CAH diagnosis uncertain at best.

One factor which may be considered in the decision to test is the ethnic/racial background of the child. While NC-CAH is common in certain ethnic groups (eg, Ashkenazi Jews), it appears to be less common to rare in African-American (AA) children. This was recently confirmed in a study of 273 patients with PP, of whom 77% were AA, but the 3 who were diagnosed with CAH (1 classic and 2 NC-CAH) were all white.[16] The investigators suggest adjusting screening protocols to reflect this finding, which would greatly reduce testing in children with PP since the majority affected at most centers in the United States are AA. This is consistent with the finding that 3 times as many AA versus white 7-year-old and 8-year-old girls have pubic hair[3], yet the accepted definition of PP is onset before age 8 regardless of racial/ethnic background.

Another concern cited as a reason to order laboratory tests for patients with PP is that the rare patient with virilization due to an adrenal or gonadal tumor might be missed.[19] These rare patients typically have many red flags which distinguish them from benign PP, including the fact that the majority will present by 5 years of age.[20] Also, the pubic hair is prominent, long, and curly; the phallus is generally enlarged; and the growth chart shows a rapid increase in both linear growth and weight gain. For virilizing adrenal tumors, evidence of glucocorticoid excess is often present. Gonadal tumors are rarely found in young children, but in males, Leydig cell tumors may present with early virilization, and a mass on 1 testis may be palpable. Females with ovarian tumors may present with both virilization and feminization as discussed in (see John S. Fuqua and Erica A. Eugster's article, "Presentation and Care for Children with Peripheral Precocious Puberty," in this issue).

IS A BONE AGE NEEDED IN PREMATURE PUBARCHE?

A BA has long been considered an important part of the evaluation of children presenting with PP. The question is how often an advanced BA will signal the presence of underlying pathology in the absence of growth acceleration or a concerning physical examination. A 2012 study of 122 patients (75% female) found that BA was greater than 2 standard deviation scores (SDSs) in 31%, PA subjects were taller, and the predicted height was at or above genetic potential. There were 11 NC-CAH patients (9%) who had earlier pubic hair, more advanced BA, lower height SDSs, lower adult height prediction, and higher adrenal androgen levels.[21]

A similar study from 2013 looked at BA in 121 5-year-old to 9-year-old patients (82% female) with PP, and similar to the previous study, found that 31% had a BA advanced by 2 or more years. Those PP patients were taller and had a greater BMI than PP patients with a normal BA, had a slightly higher mean DHEA-S, and the predicted adult height was in the normal range for all. In contrast to the 2012 study, of the 37 patients with BA advanced 2 or more years, only 1 patient (a 6 year old boy with BA of 12 years and height SDS + 3.1) was diagnosed with CAH.[22] Most but not all patients had 17-OHP levels done but the risk of missing CAH (either classic or NC-CAH) appeared to be very low in the PP patients with the most advanced BA. We would argue that for the typical scenario of 5-year-old to 9-year-old patients with PP, obtaining a BA adds cost and often anxiety but little if anything diagnostically. However, for the small subset of patients with young age at onset (outside of infancy) and evidence of virilization, BA can be a useful part of the evaluation.

SUMMARY/RECOMMENDATIONS

Most cases of PA are easily recognized on clinical grounds based on the age of onset (5–9 years for most cases), the nonprogressive or slowly progressive course, and the lack of significant growth acceleration. A careful explanation of the likely benign nature should be given to the parents, with the recommendation that testing can be deferred pending monitoring by either the endocrine provider or the primary care provider. Some may argue that failing to test on the first visit is problematic if the patient progresses and fails to return for follow-up. If the endocrine provider chooses not to schedule a follow-up visit, it is critical to detail in the letter to the referring provider (ideally with a copy to the parents) the reasons (rapid growth and/or progression) that should prompt a return visit. It is acknowledged that a very small proportion of children with early pubic hair development have serious conditions requiring testing and treatment, but those usually have red flags based on their growth and physical examination. However, continued monitoring should identify the very rare patient with another diagnosis but without red flags at the first visit. Delaying testing while reassuring parents will decrease parental anxiety, reduce unnecessary costs of care, and prevent unnecessary treatments, such as glucocorticoids for mild NC-CAH, where the benefits of treatment remain uncertain.

CLINICS CARE POINTS

- PP is a common and usually benign variant of normal puberty most often seen in 5-year-old to 9-year-old children, with about 80% being seen in females.
- In typical cases, there is pubic and/or axillary hair and an adult-type axillary odor, with slow progression, a normal growth rate, no signs of virilization, and no breast development in girls or genital enlargement in boys.
- A variant of PP is genital hair appearing in the first year of life, which is less common but also appears to be nonprogressive and benign
- While some order laboratory testing and a BA to try to rule out other diagnoses including NC-CAH and gonadal or adrenal tumors, the author recommends not testing children with PP who have no red flags at the initial visit.
- Monitoring for rapid changes in growth or physical examination findings should be done within 6 to 12 months either by the consulting or the referring provider.

DISCLOSURE

The author has no conflicts of interest to disclose.

REFERENCES

1. Utrainen P, Laakso S, Liimatta J, et al. Premature adrenarche: A common condition with variable presentation. Horm Res Paediatr 2015;83:221–3.
2. Rosenfield RL. Normal and premature adrenarche. Endocr Rev 2021;42: 783–814.
3. Biro FM, Galvez MP, Greenspan LC, et al. Pubertal assessment method and baseline characteristics in a mixed longitudinal study of girls. Pediatrics 2010; 126(3):e583.
4. Wendelin DS, Pope DN, Mallory SB. Hypertrichosis. J Am Acad Dermatol 2003; 48:161–79.
5. Kaplowitz P. Clinical characteristics of 104 children referred for evaluation of precocious puberty. J Clin Endocrinol Metab 2004;89(8):3644–50.
6. Ibanez L, Virdis R, Potau N, et al. Natural history of premature pubarche: an auxological study. J Clin Endocrinol Metab 1992;74:254–7.

7. Ibanez L, Jimenez R, de Zegher F. Early puberty-menarche after precocious pubarche: relation to prenatal growth. Pediatrics 2006;117:117–21.
8. Ibanez L, de Zegher F, Potau N. Premature pubarche, ovarian hyperandrogenism, hyperinsulinism and the polycystic ovary syndrome: from a complex constellation to a simple sequence of prenatal onset. J Endocrinol Invest 1998;21: 558–66.
9. Diamond FB, Schulman DI, Root AW. Scrotal hair in infancy. J Pediatr 1989;114: 999–1001.
10. Adams DA, Young PC, Copeland KC. Pubic hair in infancy. Am J Dis Child 1992; 146:149–51.
11. Nebesio TD, Eugster EA. Pubic hair of infancy: endocrinopathy or enigma? Pediatrics 2006;117:951–4.
12. Kaplowitz PB, Soldin SJ. Steroid profiles in serum by liquid chromatography-tandem mass spectrometry in infants with genital hair. J Pediatr Endocrinol Metab 2007;20:597–606.
13. Kaplowitz PB, Mehra R. Clinical characteristics of children referred for signs of early puberty before age 3. J Pediatr Endocrinol Metab 2015;28:1139–44.
14. Armengaud JB, Charkaluk ML, Trivin C, et al. Precocious pubarche: distinguishing late-onset congenital adrenal hyperplasia from premature adrenarche. J Clin Endocrinol Metab 2009;94(8):2835–40.
15. Bizzarri C, Crea F, Marini R, et al. Clinical features suggestive of non-classical 21-hydroxylase deficiency in children presenting with precocious pubarche. J Pediatr Endocrinol Metab 2012;25(11–12):1059–64.
16. Foster C, Diaz-Thomas A, Lahoti A. Low prevalence of organic pathology in a predominantly black population with premature adrenarche: need to stratify definitions and screening protocols. Int J Pediatr Endocrinol 2020;2020:5.
17. Wasniewska MG, Morabito LA, Baronio F, et al, Adrenal Diseases Working Group of the Italian Society for Pediatric Endocrinology and Diabetology. Growth trajectory and adult height in children with nonclassical congenital adrenal hyperplasia. Horm Res Paediatr 2020;93(3):173–81.
18. Kaplowitz PB. For premature thelarche and premature adrenarche, the case for waiting before testing. Horm Res Paediatr 2020;93:573–6.
19. Paris F, Kalfa N, Philibert P, et al. Very premature pubarche in girls is not a pubertal variant: 2 cases of adrenal tumor presenting with pubic hair before age 4. Hormones 2012;11:356–60.
20. Lee PD, Winter RJ, Green OC. Virilizing adrenocortical tumors in childhood: eight cases and a review of the literature. Pediatrics 1985 Sep;76(3):437–44.
21. Von Oettingen J, Sola Pou J, Levitsky L, et al. Clinical presentation of children with premature adrenarche. Clin Pediatr 2012 Dec;51(12):1140–9.
22. Desalvo D, Vaidyanathan P, Mehra R, Kaplowitz PB. In children with premature adrenarche, bone age advancement by 2 or more years is common and generally benign. J Pediatr Endocrinol Metab 2013;26:215–22.

Isolated Vaginal Bleeding Before the Onset of Puberty

Natalie G. Allen, MD[a],*, Paul B. Kaplowitz, MD, PhD[b]

KEYWORDS

- Premature menarche • Prepubertal vaginal bleeding • Isolated early menstruation
- Isolated vaginal bleeding • Vaginal foreign body

KEY POINTS

- Isolated vaginal bleeding before the onset of puberty typically resolves after 1 to 3 episodes.
- In most cases, watchful waiting for clinical progression is appropriate.
- Further workup should be completed when patients have persistent vaginal bleeding, other signs of puberty, or signs/symptoms of an underlying disorder.

INTRODUCTION

Isolated vaginal bleeding is an infrequent complaint in prepubertal girls that can cause significant anxiety in both the patient and caregiver. These individuals will often present to the pediatrician or family medicine provider and may additionally be evaluated by a pediatric endocrinologist or gynecologist. The differential diagnosis of vaginal bleeding without other signs of puberty includes isolated vaginal bleeding, vulvovaginitis, vaginal foreign body, benign or malignant tumor, urethral prolapse, vulvovaginal trauma, McCune-Albright syndrome, and estrogen exposure.[1] The clinician faces a dilemma of efficient use of medical resources and watchful waiting.

By definition, isolated vaginal bleeding is characterized by a single episode (including spotting) or recurrent vaginal bleeding without the presence of significant breast development. This entity is uncommon, with 1 study finding it in 2.3% of 1037 females evaluated for precocious puberty (PP),[2] and another finding it in 10% of girls aged 1 to 8 years.[3] Through the literature, isolated vaginal bleeding has been described with different terminology including premature menarche, benign prepubertal vaginal bleeding, premature isolated menses, isolated early menstruation, and isolated menarche.[2-4] While there are limited clinical data published on this entity,

[a] Department of Pediatrics, Division of Endocrinology and Diabetes, Penn State Health Milton S. Hershey Medical Center, Penn State Health, 12 Briarcrest Square, Hershey, PA 17033, USA; [b] Division of Endocrinology, Children's National Hospital, 111 Michigan Avenue Northwest, Washington, DC 20010, USA
* Corresponding author.
E-mail address: Nallen4@pennstatehealth.psu.edu

Endocrinol Metab Clin N Am 53 (2024) 211–216
https://doi.org/10.1016/j.ecl.2024.01.003

the authors will provide evidence that it is generally benign and self-limited, and thus a cost-effective approach to the workup is suitable in most cases.

BACKGROUND

Isolated vaginal bleeding was first described in the literature by Heller and colleagues[4] in 1979. They reported 4 cases of prepubertal girls with cyclical vaginal bleeding. Individuals were noted to eventually have typical timing for secondary sexual characteristics, and neither an underlying diagnosis nor explanation was noted.

A subsequent study by Murram and colleagues[5] in 1983 interviewed 12 women aged 16 to 34 years who had a previous diagnosis of isolated vaginal bleeding. All of these individuals were noted to have regular menses resuming between 10 and 14.5 years of age and several had gone on to have successful pregnancies. Attained adult height among these individuals was normal.[5]

One series published in 1989 reported on 52 girls, all aged less than 10 years, admitted to their secondary referral hospital over the course of 20 years.[6] Local lesions were the most common etiology of vaginal bleeding noted, accounting for 54% of cases with 11 cases of malignant genital tract tumors. Only 6 of 52 cases in this series were noted to be isolated vaginal bleeding. Other noted diagnoses included urethral prolapse, vulvovaginitis, and vulvar lesions.[6] In 2016, Soderstrom and colleagues[7] reported a series of 86 girls admitted to a tertiary pediatric center with vaginal bleeding. They noted 54.7% to have a local lesion, including trauma and vulvovaginitis; 18.6% were found to have a hormonal etiology; and in 26.7%, no underlying cause was noted. Note that these 2 studies focused on hospitalized cases, which the authors suggest are much more likely to uncover an underlying etiology than those referred to pediatric endocrinologists, since these referrals tend to be prompted by abnormal physical examination findings.

Another study reported on 17 individuals with isolated vaginal bleeding: 35% had only 1 episode of vaginal bleeding, 47% had 2 to 3 episodes, and 17% had 4 or more episodes. Bleeding episodes for these individuals lasted approximately 2 to 5 days.[3] Girls presented at an average age of 4 years 7 months to 8 years 2 months in reported studies.[2,3,8] Laboratory evaluation has shown a few patients with borderline elevation in baseline luteinizing hormone (LH) and rare elevations in estradiol.[8,9] Nella and colleagues[2] reported recurrence in 33% of their cohort of 24 patients, most of which were within 2 months. There were 2 individuals who experienced intermittent spotting for up to 1 year.

ETIOLOGY

Theories behind the underlying cause of isolated vaginal bleeding have included increased sensitivity of endometrial tissue to prepubertal hormone levels and transient activity of the hypothalamic–pituitary–gonadal axis.[2,3,10] Blanco-Garcia and colleagues[3] argued that given the higher incidence of female PP over male PP, ovarian tissue may have more sensitivity to gonadotropins, which may explain isolated vaginal bleeding as well as other types of isosexual precocity in females. Saggese and colleagues[10] posited that there may be sleep-related LH and follicle-stimulating hormone (FSH) rises and exaggerated transient FSH rise in girls with premature menarche.

DIFFERENTIAL DIAGNOSIS

The differential diagnosis for prepubertal vaginal bleeding includes benign isolated vaginal bleeding as well as central PP, which will typically present with progressive breast development. McCune-Albright syndrome can present with vaginal bleeding as the first pubertal sign; however, these patients should report persistence of vaginal bleeding episodes as well as subsequent progressive breast development. Classically, individuals with McCune-Albright syndrome would also have café au lait macules and fibrous dysplasia of the long bones. Hypothyroidism may also present with isolated vaginal bleeding but typically would be associated with other signs and symptoms, including slowing of growth velocity and delayed bone age.[1]

Foreign bodies are another possible diagnosis of isolated vaginal bleeding. These patients will often have a vaginal discharge and may have discomfort. A brief report of 31 girls admitted for the evaluation of vaginal discharge noted only 2 patients with foreign bodies, both of which were visible on genital examination.[11] The most commonly noted foreign bodies are toilet paper in 40% and small beads or toy parts in 25% of cases in a series of 181 patients.[12] Trauma to the genitourinary tract is considered the most common cause of vaginal bleeding and is primarily seen in the emergency department. The history may include recent injury or perineal pain and most commonly would include only 1 episode of vaginal bleeding. Vulvovaginitis is also thought to be a potential common cause of prepubertal vaginal bleeding.

Less often, patients may present with urethral prolapse or vaginal neoplasms. In the report of hospitalized patients with persistent prepubertal vaginal bleeding at a tertiary center, 5% were diagnosed with urethral prolapse and 4.4% were noted to have vaginal neoplasms.[13]

EVALUATION

History should include the heaviness of vaginal bleeding episodes and the timing of any recurrences. Critically, discussion of any other symptoms of pubertal development should take place, including breast development, axillary hair, pubic hair, growth spurt, or acne. History should also include any recent trauma, allergies, change in hygiene practices, and the use of estrogen-containing medications.

A careful physical examination is important to distinguish isolated benign vaginal bleeding from other potential causes. Initial evaluation should start with an extensive skin examination to look for café-au-lait macules and Tanner staging of breasts and pubic hair. The clinician should assess growth velocity based on growth charts. A careful genitourinary examination should assess for visible lesion or injury and estrogenization of the vaginal mucosa. Concerning history and physical examination features are noted in **Table 1**.

Bone age x-ray is a study often done in the early assessment of patients with isolated vaginal bleeding. Multiple studies have noted no advancement of bone age with benign, isolated vaginal bleeding[2,14]; however, if present, it may be a clue to true PP. Further radiographic evaluation, specifically transabdominal ultrasound and/or transperineal ultrasound, may be warranted to assess for uterine size, ovarian cysts or follicles, and possible foreign body. In a limited series, transabdominal ultrasound has noted normal uterine size for age and a lack of endometrial stripe in patients with isolated vaginal bleeding.[15] Yang and colleagues[13] found that the use of both transabdominal and transperineal ultrasound had a sensitivity of 81% and specificity of 53% in the detection of vaginal foreign bodies, with a positive predictive value of 82%. They noted that accuracy approached 100% with objects greater than 5 mm.

Laboratory assessment should be considered in patients with persistent vaginal bleeding with greater than 3 episodes, signs or symptoms suggestive of an underlying etiology, or progression of secondary sex characteristics. Diagnostic laboratory tests may include estradiol, LH, and FSH, with dehydroepiandrosterone sulfate if there is

Table 1	
History and physical examination features that should prompt further workup	
Features of History	**Possible Diagnoses**
Reported breast development	Precocious puberty
Rapid linear growth	Precocious puberty
Axillary hair, pubic hair, acne	Premature adrenarche
Recent trauma	Vaginal injury or lesion
Use of estrogen-containing medications	Estrogen exposure
Persistent bleeding>7 d	Vaginal lesion or mass
Vaginal discharge (often purulent)	Foreign body
Abdominal pain or perineal pain	Infection, mass
Fatigue, growth failure	Hypothyroidism
Features of Physical Examination	**Possible Diagnoses**
Café-au-lait spots which are unilateral	McCune-Albright syndrome
Tanner stage ≥2 breasts	Precocious puberty, estrogen exposure
Visible genitourinary lesion	Vaginal lesion or mass
Estrogenization of vaginal mucosa	Precocious puberty, estrogen exposure

pubic hair. Thyroid testing should be ordered in the rare cases with typical symptoms and clear growth deceleration. Further evaluation with gonadotropin-releasing hormone stimulation testing may be warranted if central PP is suspected and a random LH is less than 0.3 mIU/mL.

When there is suspicion of intravaginal lesions including foreign bodies, patients may require examination under anesthesia or vaginoscopy.

DISCUSSION

Isolated vaginal bleeding is a rare presentation of isosexual precocity representing approximately 5% of females presenting for care. Clinical data remain relatively limited since initial reporting on the condition.[4] Case series indicate that most patients with isolated vaginal bleeding and a normal physical examination noted resolution of symptoms within 1 to 3 episodes without further pubertal progression. Unlike patients referred to pediatric endocrine providers, case series from gynecology providers and inpatient centers show a high proportion of underlying issues, presumably because those referrals are likely driven by abnormal findings on the vaginal examination, pain, or persistent symptoms.[7,13]

There has been an ongoing discussion about the level of workup required for such cases, with some studies supporting extensive evaluation of patients both from a laboratory and radiographic perspective[1] and others considering the possibility of a more limited initial evaluation with watchful waiting.[2] Based on available data, initial watchful waiting of patients appears to be warranted in most cases. When vaginal bleeding episodes persist for greater than 3 episodes, are accompanied by other physical findings of underlying pathology, or have subsequent progressive development of secondary sex characteristics, further work up is warranted, potentially including laboratory evaluation and/or radiographic studies.

Long-term follow-up data of benign, isolated vaginal bleeding are limited, but available studies reported attainment of adult height consistent with family potential, appropriate timing of pubertal changes, regular menses, and fertility in adulthood.[3,5] Thus, reassurance of parents about the benign nature of the condition is appropriate.

SUMMARY

Isolated vaginal bleeding is a rare presentation of isosexual precocity and will typically resolve after 1 to 3 episodes without further effect on true pubertal timing. Watchful waiting and a step-by-step approach are typically appropriate in a child without breast development, pubic hair, rapid growth rate, or signs and symptoms concerning for underlying etiologies. In patients with persistent vaginal bleeding or those with other signs of puberty, further workup is needed. Transabdominal and transperineal ultrasound may be the most useful next step in those with persistent isolated vaginal bleeding, and bone age and laboratory evaluations may also be useful in selected cases.

CLINICS CARE POINTS

- Isolated vaginal bleeding will typically resolve after 1 to 3 episodes without further effect on true pubertal timing.
- Watchful waiting and a step-by-step approach are typically appropriate.
- In patients with persistent vaginal bleeding or those with other signs of puberty, further workup is needed.

DISCLOSURE

The authors have nothing to disclose.

REFERENCES

1. Dwiggins M, Gomez-Lobo V. Current review of prepubertal vaginal bleeding. Curr Opin Obstet Gynecol 2017;29(5):322–7.
2. Nella AA, Kaplowitz PB, Ramnitz MS, et al. Benign vaginal bleeding in 24 prepubertal patients: clinical, biochemical and imaging features. J Pediatr Endocrinol Metab 2014;27(9–10):821–5.
3. Blanco-Garcia M, Evain-Brion D, Roger M, et al. Isolated menses in prepubertal girls. Pediatrics 1985;76(1):43–7.
4. Heller ME, Dewhurst J, Grant DB. Premature menarche without other evidence of precocious puberty. Arch Dis Child 1979;54(6):472–5.
5. Murram D, Dewhurst J, Grant DB. Premature menarche: a follow-up study. Arch Dis Child 1983;58(2):142–3.
6. Hill NC, Oppenheimer LW, Morton KE. The aetiology of vaginal bleeding in children. A 20-year review. Br J Obstet Gynaecol 1989;96(4):467–70.
7. Söderström HF, Carlsson A, Börjesson A, et al. Vaginal Bleeding in Prepubertal Girls: Etiology and Clinical Management. J Pediatr Adolesc Gynecol 2016; 29(3):280–5.
8. Ng SM, Apperley LJ, Upradrasta S, et al. Vaginal Bleeding in Pre-pubertal Females. J Pediatr Adolesc Gynecol 2020;33(4):339–42.
9. Merckx M, Weyers S, Santegoeds R, et al. Menstrual-like vaginal bleeding in prepubertal girls: an unexplained condition. Facts Views Vis Obgyn 2011;3(4). 267-170.

10. Saggese G, Ghirri P, Del Vecchio A, et al. Gonadotropin pulsatile secretion in girls with premature menarche. Horm Res 1990;33(1):5–10.
11. Smith YR, Berman DR, Quint EH. Premenarchal Vaginal Discharge: Findings of Procedures to Rule Out Foreign Bodies. J Pediatr Adolesc Gynecol 2002;15(4): 227–30.
12. Zhang J, Zhang B, Su Y, et al. Prepubertal Vaginal Bleeding: An Inpatient Series from a Single Center in Fujian China. J Pediatr Adolesc Gynecol 2020;33(2): 120–4.
13. Yang X, Sun L, Ye J, et al. Ultrasonography in Detection of Vaginal Foreign Bodies in Girls: A Retrospective Study. J Pediatr Adolesc Gynecol 2017;30(6):620–5.
14. Ejaz S, Lane A, Wilson T. Outcome of Isolated Premature Menarche: A Retrospective and Follow-Up Study. Horm Res Paediatr 2015;84(4):217–22.
15. Pinto SM, Garden AS. Prepubertal menarche: a defined clinical entity. Am J Obstet Gynecol 2006;195(1):327–9.

Diagnosis of Central Precocious Puberty

Kanthi Bangalore Krishna, MD[a],*, Lawrence A. Silverman, MD[b]

KEYWORDS

- Precocious puberty • Gonadotropin-releasing hormone analogue
- Central precocious puberty • Peripheral precocious puberty • Bone age
- Pelvic ultrasound • Brain MRI

KEY POINTS

- A thorough history and physical examination including Tanner staging and growth assessments can guide differential diagnosis and aid in the evaluation of precocious puberty.
- Basal luteinizing hormone levels measured using a highly sensitive assay can be helpful in diagnosing central precocious puberty (CPP).
- Brain MRI is indicated with males diagnosed with CPP and females under the age of 6 with CPP. For girls with CPP between the ages of 6 and 8, shared decision making with the family should guide the need for brain imaging.
- As more information becomes available regarding the genetic etiologies of CPP, genetic testing may preclude the need for imaging studies and other hormonal testing especially in familial cases.

Gonadotropin-dependent sexual precocity, more commonly referred to as central precocious puberty (CPP), results from the premature reactivation of the hypothalamic-pituitary-gonadal (HPG) axis.[1] While data suggest that the age of onset of puberty has decreased over the past half century, clinically, the appearance of breast development before the age of 8 in girls or testicular enlargement before the age of 9 in boys is generally considered precocious.[2,3]

The mechanisms of reactivation of the HPG axis and entry into puberty are complex, with a myriad of genetic and environmental factors that regulate gonadotropin-releasing hormone (GnRH) secretion.[4] Ultimately, initiation of both normally timed and precocious puberty involves the pulsatile release of GnRH. This increased GnRH pulsatility results in the secretion of luteinizing hormone (LH) and follicle-

[a] Division of Pediatric Endocrinology and Diabetes, UPMC Childrens Hospital of Pittsburgh, 4401 Penn Avenue, Pittsburgh, PA 15224, USA; [b] Division of Pediatric Endocrinology, Goryeb Children's Hospital, Atlantic Health System, 100 Madison Avenue, Morristown, NJ 07960, USA
* Corresponding author.
E-mail address: bangalorekrishnak2@upmc.edu

Endocrinol Metab Clin N Am 53 (2024) 217–227
https://doi.org/10.1016/j.ecl.2024.02.002
0889-5529/24/© 2024 Elsevier Inc. All rights reserved.

stimulating hormone (FSH), leading to the production of gonadal sex steroids and subsequent development of secondary sexual characteristics.[5,6]

As puberty is neither a linear process nor a single event, both boys and girls may present with variations of normal pubertal development, which can be mistaken for true puberty.[7,8] Hence, it is incumbent upon the clinician to develop a paradigm in which to approach these patients from both a clinical and investigative perspective; this will lead to an accurate diagnosis which can best classify patients as normal variants or true/central or peripheral precocious puberty and develop a treatment plan as deemed necessary.

TIMING OF PUBERTY

"When twice 7 years the men engender seed and women's breasts begin to swell."[9] The timing of the onset of puberty has evolved over the past millennium, a fact well documented by the change in age of menarche over the past 2 centuries.[10,11] The classic teaching has been that the first signs of puberty, breast development, begins in girls after 8 and in boys, testicular enlargement, after 9, has evolved over the past 50 years.[12] The observations of Tanner in the 1950s, which codified pubertal development stages, harken back to original observational work from the 1920s.[7,8] While the "normal" ages of the progressive pubertal, or Tanner stages, were based on examinations of pictures of a White British population, the clinical description/changes, if not necessarily the ages, apply to all children (**Fig. 1**).

The common observation that children of different genetic backgrounds progress through puberty at different times has been well accepted over the years.[13,14] In an attempt to better codify these differences, Herman Giddens and colleagues[15] set out to define the age of onset of physical changes of puberty across races in a cross section of American girls. In an analysis of over 17,000 girls, in an office-based setting,

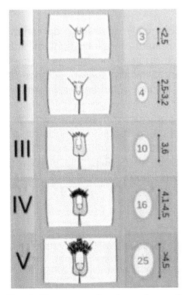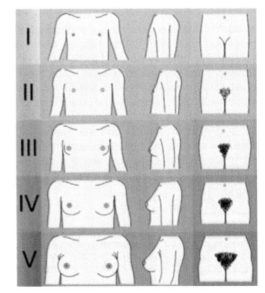

Fig. 1. Tanner staging in males and females. https://openi.nlm.nih.gov/detailedresult.php? img=PMC4478390_fnhum-09-00344-g001&req=4. (Image credit: Michał Komorniczak, 2009, CC-BY-SA 3.0. Tanner Scale Male: http://goo.gl/7cxTLM. Tanner Scale Female: http://goo.gl/haB9Cb.)

15% of African American girls and 5% of White girls were noted to have breast development before the age of 8, with a mean age of 8.87 years and 9.96, respectively. In this cohort, the mean age of menarche was 12.16 years in African American girls and 12.88 in White girls. While there are well-described concerns with the methods employed by this study, including the lack of hormonal testing, it did speak to the well-observed trend noted by primary care pediatricians and endocrinologists alike.[15] A subsequent, albeit smaller but perhaps more powerful, observational study about the timing of puberty came out of the Breast Cancer and the Environment Research Program.[3] In this study, a team of researchers were specifically trained, and cross tested, to evaluate the presence of breast development by palpation in girls over time at 3 distinct centers in 4 distinct genetic/ethnic cohorts: African American, Hispanic, white non-Hispanic, and Asian, The median ages of T2 breast development were 8.8, 9.3, 9.7, and 9.7 years, respectively. More importantly, 18% of African American and 3% of White girls had stage 2 breast development by age 7, and 22% and 5% by age 8 (**Fig. 2**). The 14.2% variance in timing was accounted for by weight/body mass index (BMI), while only 4.4% was accounted for by race. When this cohort was followed to document age of menarche, the median age of menarche for the entire group was 12.25 years: African American 12.0, Hispanic 11.83, Asian 12.75, and White 12.67 years. A correlation existed between BMI and age of menarche, with an inverse correlation between higher BMI and earlier age of first menstrual cycle.

Interestingly, those girls with the earlier timing of B2 had a slower progression of puberty, with those with B2 earlier than 8.5 years having a median tempo of 42 months to menarche, while in those with B2 after 10.5 years it was 25 months to first menses.[14]

CLINICAL EVALUATION

As with the approach to any patient, a thorough history involves focus upon timing and sequence of initial changes; timing of puberty in parents, grandparents, and siblings; general health; medications; and exposures. Other aspects including birth history, length and weight, the presence of small for gestational age[16] or prematurity, and central nervous system (CNS) insult at birth or later are informative.[17] A history of gelastic seizures may point to the presence of a hypothalamic hamartoma. A careful history to rule out exposure to hormone-containing creams or medications; exposure to lavender or tea tree oil, which can activate the E2 receptor[18]; or disease states such as congenital adrenal hyperplasia or other autonomous endocrine function may be pertinent. Data points from the growth curve can also provide further clarification of the

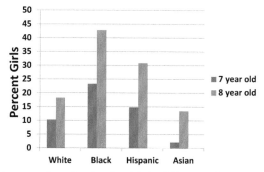

Fig. 2. Breast development by palpation in girls in different ethnic groups. (*Adapted from* Biro F, Greenspan L, Galvez M, Pinney S, Teitelbaum S, Windham G, et al. Onset of Breast Development in a Longitudinal Cohort. Pediatrics. 2013;132(6): 1019–1027.)

timing of a growth acceleration, which is generally observed in girls after Tanner 2 breast development and in boys at Tanner 3 to 4. As the first clinical signs of puberty are related to gonadal sex steroid production, a careful physical examination can help differentiate true puberty from variations in development (adrenarche and thelarche). Usually girls present with breast development, while testicular enlargement in a boy is the first finding,[7] with volume being greater than 3 mL or length being 2.5 cm or more. As originally described,[8] Tanner 2 breast development involves the present of a breast bud with elevation of the papilla and enlargement of the areola. The presence of pubic hair (Tanner stage 2 or more) does not necessarily indicate gonadal steroid secretion, that is, gonadarche, since pubarche may be secondary to adrenarche. It is not uncommon for this process to precede true central puberty.

A frequent clinical conundrum is the need to differentiate, on physical examination, between adipose chest tissue (adipomastia/lipomastia) and true breast budding in girls. Perhaps the most challenging patients are those girls who are overweight. On examination, one can attempt to discern if there is tissue directly below the nipple as the first breast buds are subareolar. In contrast, depression of the nipple on palpation, with no tissue directly under the nipple but surrounding the finger, forming the so-called "doughnut sign" may be informative. While frequently used to differentiate gynecomastia from lipomastia in overweight boys, it can be employed in peripubertal girls. Similarly, if one "pinches" the area surround the nipple, a true breast bud will be discernible between the fingers; this is unlikely in the presence of adipose tissue alone. The presence of a breast bud within significant adipose tissue in the chest is not uncommon. Some posit that this can be secondary to the effect of local aromatase activity present in the adipose tissue.[19]

For boys, staging of penis and pubic hair development plus testicular volume is necessary. Accurate measurement of either testicular volume using an orchidometer (**Fig. 3**) or testicular length is essential.

Other aspects of the physical examination that require specific focus include the skin; café au lait spots can point to either McCune-Albright syndrome or neurofibromatosis type 1. The melanocytic macules of Peutz-Jeghers syndrome could point to the presence of a sex cord tumor causing gonadotropin-independent (peripheral) sexual precocity.

LABORATORY EVALUATION

While a differential diagnosis is based on a thorough history and physical examination, laboratory evaluation is necessary to diagnose precocious puberty and the possible etiology.

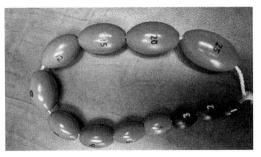

Fig. 3. Orchidometer showing representative testicular volumes ranging from prepubertal (1 ml–3 ml) and pubertal testes (4 ml to 25 ml).

Circulating gonadotropin and sex steroid concentrations assess the status of the HPG axis.[20,21] Historically, the established gold standard was the LH and FSH response to a standard bolus of native GnRH. However native GnRH is no longer available in the United States, and most stimulation tests are now performed with the GnRH analogue (GnRHa) leuprolide acetate, a synthetic nonapeptide with much greater potency. Due to the pharmacodynamic differences between these 2 medications, the timing and peak values of FSH and LH levels are different. Following native GnRH administration, LH levels peak after 20 to 40 minutes, followed by a decline in values compared with leuprolide acetate, which can similarly stimulate LH to peak as early as 30 minutes to 4 hours followed by sustained LH elevation.[22–24]

The development of highly sensitive and pediatric-specific gonadotropin assays has added to our diagnostic armamentarium. With the development of more sensitive assays, many practitioners have come to rely on the utility of random LH levels, with a cutoff of 0.3 to 0.5 IU/L.[25] While this cutoff value has high sensitivity greater than 90%, it has a relatively low specificity, as a percentage of girls with true central puberty will have a random LH lower than the aforementioned cutoff values.[21,26] The lower limit of detection for most ultrasensitive immunochemiluminescent assays (ICMA) is ≤ 0.1 mIU/mL.[26–28] Elevated basal LH levels show high sensitivity and specificity for boys when a high-quality ICMA is used.[29] Different cut-points need to be used to interpret LH concentrations in girls under 2 years of age because LH concentrations may normally be higher (minipuberty of infancy); CPP may frequently be misdiagnosed during this phase of development.[30]

As the short-acting GnRHas have greater affinity for the GnRH receptor than native GnRH, they lead to both an immediate release of LH and FSH from pituitary stores as well as transcription, translation, and production of LH and FSH, with subsequent spikes in sex hormones.[31] Hence, evaluating a 1-hour to 2-hour post-stimulation LH and FSH, as well as an 18-hour to 24-hour sex steroid level, has led to development of a modified stimulation test.[32] Not infrequently, there can be a less than pubertal peak LH, with a markedly pubertal sex hormone level the next day; this stimulation test does provide significant utility in confirming the presence of central puberty.[31] Both short-acting, aqueous leuprolide acetate and triptorelin have been used for this purpose[33]

As highly sensitive and specific assays have been developed, random sex hormone levels can define the presence of biochemical puberty. These levels will not differentiate gonadotropin-dependent (central) versus gonadotropin-independent (peripheral) puberty, thus the presence of a pubertal LH is necessary to confirm the diagnosis. Given the minor structural differences between steroid molecules, immunoassays measuring sex steroids are prone to cross-reactivity. Most commercial immunoassays for estradiol are designed to measure estradiol within the "normal adult female" reference range and therefore have low sensitivity and specificity to quantify the low concentrations (<30 pg/mL) typically found in prepubertal children. More recently, methods utilizing liquid chromatographic separation followed by tandem mass spectrometry (LC-MS/MS) have been developed. Serum testosterone is also best measured using LC-MS/MS technology to limit cross-reactivity.

In children with precocious pubarche, the measurement of adrenal steroids may be necessary to help distinguish between peripheral precocity and benign premature adrenarche. Children with premature adrenarche can have mild elevation in adrenal hormones.[34] An early-morning 17-hydroxyprogesterone value greater than 200 ng/dL (6 nmol/L) has a high sensitivity and specificity for nonclassic congenital adrenal hyperplasia secondary to 21-hydroxylase deficiency. An adrenocorticotropic hormone stimulation test may still be needed to confirm the diagnosis.[35,36]

A thyroid-stimulating hormone concentration should be measured if chronic primary hypothyroidism is suspected as the underlying cause for the sexual precocity.[37,38]

IMAGING STUDIES
Bone Age

The assessment of skeletal maturation is based on an X ray of the left hand and wrist, most commonly using the Greulich and Pyle method in which the patient's bone age radiograph is compared with an atlas of radiographs from children of known ages.[39] Another method which is used less frequently is the Tanner-Whitehouse 2 method, in which 20 different hand and wrist bones are individually scored. Additional factors such as other hormones, obesity, genetics, nutritional status, various disease states, and certain medications can influence the rate of epiphyseal maturation[40] .[41] Using the tables of Bayley and Pinneau, a median predicted adult height (PAH) may be calculated and compared to the patient's target height based on the mid parental height.

Although the PAH using the bone age may help guide treatment decisions,[42] there is a tendency to overestimate adult height.[43] As the use of automated measurement systems with artificial intelligence has increased, previous limitations were apparently in part due to intraobserver and interobserver variability.[44,45]

Pelvic Ultrasound

During puberty, increased gonadotropin secretion promotes ovarian growth and increased estradiol secretion. Concomitantly, pelvic ultrasound shows increased uterine size and ovarian volume. In general, uterine lengths greater than 3.5 to 4 cm and ovarian volumes greater than 2 mL are consistent with puberty.[46] However, overlap of these measurements between prepubertal and early pubertal size may confound interpretation.[47,48] The use of Doppler ultrasound to assess utero-ovarian blood flow may provide helpful information.[49–52]

Brain MRI

Brain MRI defines brain and pituitary anatomy. Due to the higher probability of finding a CNS anomaly, most studies recommend a contrast-enhanced, pituitary-focused, brain MRI for all males with CPP[53] and for females with onset of secondary sexual characteristics before 6 years of age because of higher rates of CNS abnormalities in these groups of patients.[25] Females with CPP onset between 6 and 8 years of age may not need the MRI if there is no clinical evidence of CNS pathology and if there is a family history of earlier pubertal onset, or if the child has an increased BMI.[54] The low prevalence of CNS lesions in females with the onset of puberty after age 6 years does challenge the need for all females in this age group to have imaging,[55,56] and hence MRI should be limited to high-risk individuals.[57] In a 2018 meta-analysis,[58] the prevalence of intracranial lesions was 3% among females presenting with CPP after 6 years of age, compared with 25% among those presenting before 6 years. Current guidelines recommend that in otherwise asymptomatic girls with CPP, a discussion must occur with the parents regarding the pros and cons of brain imaging to assist in informed decision-making.[25,59,60] While brain MRIs are recommended for all boys presenting with CPP, 1 study found that these rates may be overestimated and none of the identified lesions necessitated treatment, suggesting the need to globally reevaluate the prevalence of pathologic brain lesions among boys with CPP.[61]

Genetic Testing

CPP can be sporadic or familial.[62] The past 15 years have seen a marked increase in the discovery and characterization of both normally functioning genes and pathologic variants associated with CPP. Genome-wide association studies and other technologies have further increased the discovery of genetic loci associated with pubertal timing.[63] Among children with familial CPP, those with defects in MKRN3 and DLK1(both paternally expressed imprinted genes) do not have structural lesions in brain MRI.[64] It is likely that with the expanded use of genetic tools in the clinic, understanding of what truly controls the onset of puberty will further expand and point not only to what controls the timing but also the tempo of pubertal progression. Perhaps in the not-too-distant future, true genotype/phenotype correlations will help drive therapeutic considerations.[63]

SUMMARY

While the mechanisms underlying the control of the onset of puberty are yet to be fully comprehended, there has been an evolution in both the diagnostic and therapeutic approach to such patients. The astute clinician will recognize the need for evaluation based on signs and symptoms encountered and only then should employ the most appropriate focused approach to define if true puberty is present. While the approach can be algorithm driven, there is not a "one-size-fits-all" paradigm, and one should choose the most informative and specific tests for the clinical situation at hand.

CLINICS CARE POINTS

- Re-emergence of GnRH pulsatility results in the anterior pituitary secretion of LH and FSH, leading to the production of gonadal sex steroids and subsequent development of secondary sexual characteristics.
- Although GnRH stimulation testing has been considered the gold standard for the diagnosis of CPP, a basal ultrasensitive LH level of greater than 0.2 IU/L may be used for the diagnosis of CPP.
- Pelvic ultrasound has been found to be a useful adjunct to support the diagnosis of CPP over other forms of puberty in girls, especially when laboratory studies are equivocal.
- Guidelines regarding the need for brain imaging have been debated. Brain imaging is recommended in the evaluation of all boys with CPP and in girls under the age of 6 years. For girls older than age 6, shared decision-making after assessing the risk for neurologic manifestations, reviewing the family history, assessing the tempo of puberty as well as the risk for the procedure itself, is recommended.

DISCLOSURE

K. Bangalore Krishna has no relevant disclosures to this article. L.A. Silverman has been a consultant for Tolmar, a Data and Safety Monitoring Board member for Myovant, and with the Speaker's Bureau for Abbvie.

REFERENCES

1. Apter D, Butzow TL, Laughlin GA, et al. Gonadotropin-releasing hormone pulse generator activity during pubertal transition in girls: pulsatile and diurnal patterns of circulating gonadotropins. J Clin Endocrinol Metab 1993;76(4):940–9.
2. Biro FM, Pajak A, Wolff MS, et al. Age of Menarche in a Longitudinal US Cohort. J Pediatr Adolesc Gynecol 2018;31(4):339–45.
3. Biro F, Greenspan L, Galvez M, et al. Onset of Breast Development in a Longitudinal Cohort. Pediatrics 2013;132(6).

4. Garcia JP, Guerriero KA, Keen KL, et al. Kisspeptin and Neurokinin B Signaling Network Underlies the Pubertal Increase in GnRH Release in Female Rhesus Monkeys. Endocrinology 2017;158(10):3269–80.

5. Fuqua JS, Eugster EA. History of Puberty: Normal and Precocious. Horm Res Paediatr 2022;95(6):568–78.

6. Grumbach MM. The neuroendocrinology of human puberty revisited. Horm Res 2002;57(Suppl 2):2–14.

7. Marshall WA, Tanner JM. Variations in the pattern of pubertal changes in boys. Arch Dis Child 1970;45(239):13–23.

8. Marshall WA, Tanner JM. Variations in pattern of pubertal changes in girls. Arch Dis Child 1969;44(235):291–303.

9. Aristotle Cresswell R, Schneider JG. Aristotle's History of animals. In ten booksix. London: H. G. Bohn; 1862. p. 326.

10. Liu W, Yan X, Li C, et al. A secular trend in age at menarche in Yunnan Province, China: a multiethnic population study of 1,275,000 women. BMC Publ Health 2021;21(1):1890.

11. Cabrera SM, Bright GM, Frane JW, et al. Age of thelarche and menarche in contemporary US females: a cross-sectional analysis. J Pediatr Endocrinol Metab 2014;27(1–2):47–51.

12. Eckert-Lind C, Busch AS, Petersen JH, et al. Worldwide Secular Trends in Age at Pubertal Onset Assessed by Breast Development Among Girls: A Systematic Review and Meta-analysis. JAMA Pediatr 2020;174(4):e195881.

13. Biro FM, McMahon RP, Striegel-Moore R, et al. Impact of timing of pubertal maturation on growth in black and white female adolescents: The National Heart, Lung, and Blood Institute Growth and Health Study. J Pediatr 2001;138(5): 636–43.

14. Biro FM, Galvez MP, Greenspan LC, et al. Pubertal assessment method and baseline characteristics in a mixed longitudinal study of girls. Pediatrics 2010; 126(3):e583–90.

15. Herman-Giddens ME, Slora EJ, Wasserman RC, et al. Secondary sexual characteristics and menses in young girls seen in office practice: a study from the Pediatric Research in Office Settings network. Pediatrics 1997;99(4):505–12.

16. Ibanez L, Ferrer A, Marcos MV, et al. Early puberty: rapid progression and reduced final height in girls with low birth weight. Pediatrics 2000;106(5):E72.

17. Partsch CJ, Sippell WG. Pathogenesis and epidemiology of precocious puberty. Effects of exogenous oestrogens. Hum Reprod Update 2001;7(3):292–302.

18. Henley DV, Lipson N, Korach KS, et al. Prepubertal gynecomastia linked to lavender and tea tree oils. N Engl J Med 2007;356(5):479–85.

19. Carlson L, Flores Poccia V, Sun BZ, et al. Early breast development in overweight girls: does estrogen made by adipose tissue play a role? Int J Obes 2019;43(10): 1978–87.

20. Carel JC, Léger J. Clinical practice. Precocious puberty. N Engl J Med 2008; 358(22):2366–77.

21. Carel JC, Eugster EA, Rogol A, et al. Consensus statement on the use of gonadotropin-releasing hormone analogs in children. Pediatrics 2009;123(4): e752–62.

22. Chin VL, Cai Z, Lam L, et al. Evaluation of puberty by verifying spontaneous and stimulated gonadotropin values in girls. J Pediatr Endocrinol Metab 2015; 28(3–4):387–92.

23. Ibanez L, Potau N, Zampolli M, et al. Use of leuprolide acetate response patterns in the early diagnosis of pubertal disorders: comparison with the gonadotropin-releasing hormone test. J Clin Endocrinol Metab 1994;78(1):30–5.

24. Houk CP, Kunselman AR, Lee PA. The diagnostic value of a brief GnRH analogue stimulation test in girls with central precocious puberty: a single 30-minute post-stimulation LH sample is adequate. J Pediatr Endocrinol Metab 2008;21(12): 1113–8.

25. Bangalore Krishna K, Fuqua JS, Rogol AD, et al. Use of Gonadotropin-Releasing Hormone Analogs in Children: Update by an International Consortium. Horm Res Paediatr 2019;91(6):357–72.

26. Neely EK, Hintz RL, Wilson DM, et al. Normal ranges for immunochemiluminometric gonadotropin assays. J Pediatr 1995;127(1):40–6.

27. Neely EK, Silverman LA, Geffner ME, et al. Random unstimulated pediatric luteinizing hormone levels are not reliable in the assessment of pubertal suppression during histrelin implant therapy. Int J Pediatr Endocrinol 2013;2013(1):20.

28. Martinez-Aguayo A, Hernández MI, Capurro T, et al. Leuprolide acetate gonadotrophin response patterns during female puberty. Clin Endocrinol 2010;72(4): 489–95.

29. Howard SR. Interpretation of reproductive hormones before, during and after the pubertal transition-Identifying health and disordered puberty. Clin Endocrinol 2021;95(5):702–15.

30. Bizzarri C, Spadoni GL, Bottaro G, et al. The response to gonadotropin releasing hormone (GnRH) stimulation test does not predict the progression to true precocious puberty in girls with onset of premature thelarche in the first three years of life. J Clin Endocrinol Metab 2014;99(2):433–9.

31. Sathasivam A, Garibaldi L, Shapiro S, et al. Leuprolide stimulation testing for the evaluation of early female sexual maturation. Clin Endocrinol 2010;73(3):375–81.

32. Garibaldi LR, Aceto T Jr, Weber C, et al. The relationship between luteinizing hormone and estradiol secretion in female precocious puberty: evaluation by sensitive gonadotropin assays and the leuprolide stimulation test. J Clin Endocrinol Metab 1993;76(4):851–6.

33. Strich D, Kvatinsky N, Hirsch HJ, et al. Triptorelin depot stimulation test for central precocious puberty. J Pediatr Endocrinol Metab 2013;26(7–8):631–4.

34. Rosenfield RL. Normal and Premature Adrenarche. Endocr Rev 2021;42(6): 783–814.

35. Chesover AD, Millar H, Sepiashvili L, et al. Screening for Nonclassic Congenital Adrenal Hyperplasia in the Era of Liquid Chromatography-Tandem Mass Spectrometry. J Endocr Soc 2020;4(2):bvz030.

36. Witchel SF, Pinto B, Burghard AC, et al. Update on adrenarche. Curr Opin Pediatr 2020;32(4):574–81.

37. Reddy P, Tiwari K, Kulkarni A, et al. Van Wyk Grumbach Syndrome: A Rare Consequence of Hypothyroidism. Indian J Pediatr 2018;85(11):1028–30.

38. Baranowski E, Hogler W. An unusual presentation of acquired hypothyroidism: the Van Wyk-Grumbach syndrome. Eur J Endocrinol 2012;166(3):537–42.

39. Greulich WWPS. Radiographic atlas of skeletal development of the hand and wrist. 2nd edition. CA, USA: Stanford University Press; 1999.

40. Klein KO, Newfield RS, Hassink SG. Bone maturation along the spectrum from normal weight to obesity: a complex interplay of sex, growth factors and weight gain. J Pediatr Endocrinol Metab 2016;29(3):311–8.

41. Oh MS, Kim S, Lee J, et al. Factors associated with Advanced Bone Age in Overweight and Obese Children. Pediatr Gastroentero 2020;23(1):89–97.

42. Bar A, Linder B, Sobel EH, et al. Bayley-Pinneau Method of Height Prediction in Girls with Central Precocious Puberty - Correlation with Adult Height. J Pediatr Urol 1995;126(6):955–8.
43. Eitel KB, Eugster EA. Differences in Bone Age Readings between Pediatric Endocrinologists and Radiologists. Endocr Pract 2020;26(3):328–31.
44. Wang X, Zhou B, Gong P, et al. Artificial Intelligence-Assisted Bone Age Assessment to Improve the Accuracy and Consistency of Physicians With Different Levels of Experience. Frontiers in Pediatrics 2022;10.
45. Thodberg HH, Thodberg B, Ahlkvist J, et al. Autonomous artificial intelligence in pediatric radiology: the use and perception of BoneXpert for bone age assessment. Pediatr Radiol 2022;52(7):1338–46.
46. de Vries L, Horev G, Schwartz M, et al. Ultrasonographic and clinical parameters for early differentiation between precocious puberty and premature thelarche. Eur J Endocrinol 2006;154(6):891–8.
47. Sathasivam A, Rosenberg HK, Shapiro S, et al. Pelvic ultrasonography in the evaluation of central precocious puberty: comparison with leuprolide stimulation test. J Pediatr 2011;159(3):490–5.
48. Lee SH, Joo EY, Lee JE, et al. The Diagnostic Value of Pelvic Ultrasound in Girls with Central Precocious Puberty. Chonnam Med J 2016;52(1):70–4.
49. Battaglia C, Mancini F, Regnani G, et al. Pelvic ultrasound and color Doppler findings in different isosexual precocities. Ultrasound Obstet Gynecol 2003;22(3):277–83.
50. Long MG, Boultbee JE, Hanson ME, et al. Doppler time velocity waveform studies of the uterine artery and uterus. Br J Obstet Gynaecol 1989;96(5):588–93.
51. Paesano PL, Colantoni C, Mora S, et al. Validation of an Accurate and Noninvasive Tool to Exclude Female Precocious Puberty: Pelvic Ultrasound With Uterine Artery Pulsatility Index. Am J Roentgenol 2019;213(2):451–7.
52. Cheuiche AV, Moro C, Lucena IRS, et al. Accuracy of doppler assessment of the uterine arteries for the diagnosis of pubertal onset in girls: a scoping review. Sci Rep 2023;13(1):5791.
53. Topor LS, Bowerman K, Machan JT, et al. Central precocious puberty in Boston boys: A 10-year single center experience. PLoS One 2018;13(6):e0199019.
54. Pedicelli S, Alessio P, Scire G, et al. Routine screening by brain magnetic resonance imaging is not indicated in every girl with onset of puberty between the ages of 6 and 8 years. J Clin Endocrinol Metab 2014;99(12):4455–61.
55. Kaplowitz PB. Do 6-8 year old girls with central precocious puberty need routine brain imaging? Int J Pediatr Endocrinol 2016;2016:9.
56. Mogensen SS, Aksglaede L, Mouritsen A, et al. Pathological and Incidental Findings on Brain MRI in a Single-Center Study of 229 Consecutive Girls with Early or Precocious Puberty. PLoS One 2012;7(1).
57. Hansen AB, Renault CH, Wojdemann D, et al. Neuroimaging in 205 consecutive Children Diagnosed with Central Precocious Puberty in Denmark. Pediatr Res 2023;93(1):125–30.
58. Cantas-Orsdemir S, Garb JL, Allen HF. Prevalence of cranial MRI findings in girls with central precocious puberty: a systematic review and meta-analysis. J Pediatr Endocrinol Metab 2018;31(7):701–10.
59. Kim SH, Ahn MB, Cho WK, et al. Findings of Brain Magnetic Resonance Imaging in Girls with Central Precocious Puberty Compared with Girls with Chronic or Recurrent Headache. J Clin Med 2021;10(10).
60. Eugster EA. Update on Precocious Puberty in Girls. J Pediatr Adol Gynec 2019;32(5):455–9.

61. Yoon JS, So CH, Lee HS, et al. The prevalence of brain abnormalities in boys with central precocious puberty may be overestimated. PLoS One 2018;13(4).
62. de Vries L, Kauschansky A, Shohat M, et al. Familial central precocious puberty suggests autosomal dominant inheritance. J Clin Endocrinol Metab 2004;89(4): 1794–800.
63. Moise-Silverman J, Silverman LA. A review of the genetics and epigenetics of central precocious puberty. Front Endocrinol 2022;13:1029137.
64. Tajima T. Genetic causes of central precocious puberty. Clin Pediatr Endocrinol 2022;31(3):101–9.

Treatment of Central Precocious Puberty with a Focus on Girls

Kanthi Bangalore Krishna, MD[a],*, Karen O. Klein, MD[b],
Erica A. Eugster, MD[c]

KEYWORDS

- Precocious puberty • Gonadotropin-releasing hormone analog (GnRHa)
- Central precocious puberty • Predicted adult height • Bone age

KEY POINTS

- An increasing number of gonadotropin-releasing hormone analogs (GnRHas) are available for treatment of central precocious puberty.
- GnRHas are safe and efficacious to suppress puberty and preserve adult height.
- Treatment monitoring, duration, and outcomes are discussed.

Central precocious puberty (CPP) refers to early maturation of the hypothalamic-pituitary-gonadal axis (HPG) axis with subsequent secondary sexual development.[1] The age of thelarche has declined in the past few decades but not the age of menarche.[2] This is important when assessing girls who present with breast development between 6 and 8 years because not all of them will need treatment.[3] The decision for treatment depends on age, bone age (BA), rate of pubertal progression, height velocity, psychosocial factors, and predicted adult height (PAH), with the caveat that height predictions are not precise and BA interpretation is variable.[4] A subset of children have a slowly progressive form of CPP and do not benefit from intervention in terms of final adult height.[5]

The primary goals of treatment in CPP are to align pubertal progression with peers, prevent menarche in very young girls, and preserve adult height. Gonadotropin-releasing hormone analog (GnRHa) treatment is very efficacious toward these goals.[6] However, there is a demonstrable lack of randomized prospective studies in CPP, and the effect of GnRHas on adult height is multifactorial (chronologic age, pubertal stage, skeletal maturation, and tempo of puberty). Girls who start GnRHas before the age of

[a] Division of Pediatric Endocrinology and Diabetes, UPMC Childrens Hospital of Pittsburgh, Pittsburgh, PA 15090, USA; [b] Division of Pediatric Endocrinology and Diabetes, University of California, Rady Children's Hospital, 9500 Gilman Drive, #La Jolla, San Diego, CA 92093, USA; [c] Division of Pediatric Endocrinology, 705 Riley Hospital Drive, Indianapolis, IN 46202, USA
* Corresponding author. 4401 Penn Avenue, Pittsburgh, PA 15224.
E-mail address: bangalorekrishnak2@upmc.edu

Endocrinol Metab Clin N Am 53 (2024) 229–238
https://doi.org/10.1016/j.ecl.2024.01.004
0889-8529/24/© 2024 Elsevier Inc. All rights reserved.
endo.theclinics.com

6 years derive the most benefit from treatment, whereas the response varies from little to as much as 10 cm gains for those treated after 6 years.[7]

Adolescents with early menarche have higher rates of depression and antisocial behavior, persisting into adulthood.[8] Early menarche is also associated with an increased likelihood of teenage pregnancy and childbearing, sexual and physical assault, and reduced rates of high school graduation.[9] To date, there is no convincing evidence that these observations are applicable to children with CPP, and there are no studies that show whether therapy with GnRHas mitigates these effects. This is an area in which more research is needed.

GONADOTROPIN-RELEASING HORMONE ANALOGS

The discovery that a continuous high concentration of GnRH causes a paradoxic suppression of the HPG axis forms the basis for the GnRHas, the development of which revolutionized the treatment of CPP worldwide.[10] All are produced through minor chemical modifications of the native GnRH molecule, which greatly prolong its half-life. Initial GnRHas required daily subcutaneous or intranasal administration, with the most widely used subsequent preparation consisting of monthly weight-based dosing of intramuscular depot leuprolide. However, in the last 15 years, several extended-release GnRHa formulations have emerged that are available in a single dosage regardless of weight[4] (**Fig. 1**).

The first of these was the subcutaneous histrelin implant, which is inserted in the upper arm and contains 50 mg of drug that is released at a rate of 65 mcg per day.[11] Although the histrelin implant is marketed for annual use, it lasts for at least 2 years.[12,13] In fact, there are reports of patients being lost to follow-up who have implants in situ that are apparently causing continued suppression of puberty over many years. One potential downside to prolonged use of a single implant is the propensity for the device to break during explantation, which rarely may require ultrasound to identify retained fragments. Additional longer acting GnRHa preparations consist of either 3- or 6-monthly injectables. These include 3-monthly leuprolide, 6-monthly triptorelin, 6-monthly subcutaneous leuprolide, and 6-monthly intramuscular leuprolide. A 12-monthly injectable GnRHa formulation is currently under investigation. Some depot forms approved for intramuscular use have been administered subcutaneously with excellent success.

GnRHas are remarkably efficacious in regard to biochemical and clinical suppression, with extremely rare reports of treatment failure. The degree of biochemical suppression, determined by peak-stimulated leutinizing hormone (LH) concentrations, is somewhat variable across different doses and preparations. One consistent finding has been a lesser degree of LH suppression with the 11.25 mg 3-monthly depot

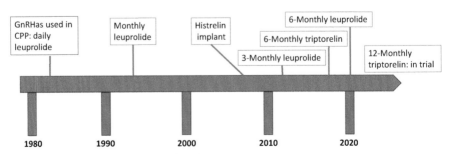

Fig. 1. Timeline of GnRHa approval in the USA

leuprolide compared with the 22.5 and 30 mg doses.[14,15] The definition of biochemical suppression is most often defined as a peak-stimulated LH level less than 4 IU/L. Less than 100% suppression to this level at 3 and 6 months was also observed in a meta-analysis of the 11.25 mg 3-monthly triptorelin formulation.[16] The 6-monthly intramuscular 22.5 mg triptorelin preparation achieved 93% suppression at 6 months and 98% at 12 months,[17] whereas the 45 mg 6-monthly subcutaneous leuprolide resulted in 87% and 86% suppression at 6 and 12 months, respectively.[18] Intramuscular 45 mg 6-monthly depot leuprolide achieved 86.7% suppression at 6 months,[19] whereas the histrelin implant causes continued very low levels of LH throughout the years of treatment.[11] However, there is no evidence that these minor differences in biochemical suppression are clinically significant because the response to treatment as evidenced by pubertal staging, height velocity, and rates of BA advancement has been excellent in all studies and almost all patients.[20] To date, there has been no head-to-head comparison of the different GnRHas. In the clinical setting, all of the therapeutic options are considered equally effective, with individual treatment decisions dictated by parental preference and/or insurance coverage (**Table 1**).

GnRHas are extremely safe. The most commonly reported adverse events are injection site reactions, which are usually mild.[21] An uncommon but more serious side effect is the development of sterile abscesses, which have been reported in patients treated with injections and the histrelin implant.[22] Girls may experience one or two episodes of vaginal bleeding after treatment initiation due to either the transient increase in HPG axis activity or the rapid withdrawal of estrogen.[23] Other minor short-term side effects have included headaches, hot flashes, and mood swings. Rare reports of hypersensitivity reactions, seizures, slipped capital femoral epiphysis, pseudotumor cerebri, hypertension, and anaphylaxis have also been reported, although the causal nature of these events has not been established.[24] Efficacy and safety in very young children is equivalent to that seen in older patients.[25]

Height velocity can significantly decline during treatment with GnRHa in some children, particularly in those with a markedly advanced BA.[26] The use of other height augmenting medications, including recombinant human growth hormone,[27] stanozolol,[28] and oxandrolone,[29] has been explored but none is routinely recommended.[30] Large, rigorously conducted randomized controlled trials are needed in order to optimize growth in girls with idiopathic CPP between the ages of 6 and 8 years.

Monitoring

The efficacy of treatment is monitored by clinical pubertal progression, ultrasensitive LH, follicle-stimulating hormone (FSH), sex hormones, BA, PAH changes, and patient satisfaction. Many clinicians forgo blood tests if clinical indices are reassuring. Treatment decisions need to be individualized, and no one variable alone predicts adequate treatment response.[31] Clinical trials for the available GnRHas report a range of response in each of the variables.[14,18,32,33]

Pubertal examination and patient satisfaction are important in monitoring treatment efficacy. Previously stimulated breast tissue may stabilize or become softer and smaller but should not progress. Mood changes reported before treatment often resolve. A change in mood or behavior in the week before an injection may indicate the rare need to shorten the treatment interval to maintain adequate suppression. However, there are no rigorous data to support this practice.

A peak GnRHa-stimulated LH level less than 4 IU/L has been used to define biochemical suppression in most studies.[4,33] A random ultrasensitive LH less than 0.6 IU/L has also been proposed to define biochemical suppression, but higher values do not necessarily indicate that escape from suppression has occurred.[33,34]

Table 1
Characteristics of different gonadotropin-releasing hormone analog preparations

Brand	Lupron Ped	Supprelin	Triptodur	Eligard/Fensolvi
GnRHa	Leuprolide	Histrelin	Triptorelin	Leuprolide
Dose	7.5, 11.25, 15 mg monthly 11.25 and 30 mg 3 mo 45 mg 6 mo	50 mg 65 mcg/d	22.5 mg	45 mg
Frequency	Every 1–6 mo	Every 1–2 y	Every 6 mo	Every 6 mo
Route	Intramuscular injection[a]	Surgical implant	Intramuscular injection	Subcutaneous injection
Data available	30 y for monthly	16 y	6 y	3 y
Injection volume (mL)	1.0–1.5	NA	2.0	0.4
Needle size (gauge)	23	NA	21	18
Needle length (inch)	1.5	NA	1.5	0.6
% below primary study stimulated LH threshold	91% LH < 1.75 in monthly 79% LH < 4 11.25 mg 3 mo 95% LH < 4 30 mg 3 mo 87% LH < 4 45 mg 6 mo	100% LH < 4	93% LH < 5	87% LH < 4
FDA approval	1 m: 1993 3 m: 2011	2007	2017	2020

[a] Anecdotal evidence suggests that subcutaneous administration suppresses similarly.

Because estradiol and testosterone levels are limited by the sensitivity of the assays, low levels of these hormones are not particularly informative. In contrast, higher levels of sex steroids are suggestive of a lack of suppression. Peak-stimulated LH levels should be suppressed by 1 month after treatment initiation no matter which preparation is used.

Adequate treatment results in a decline in rate of change in BA. For example, BA is usually advancing more than 1 year per year of chronologic age before treatment and should slow from that point. The best treatment responses include BA progression less than 1 year per year of CA. However, the decline in BA/chronological age (CA) is nonlinear, and larger declines are seen in the first 18 months of treatment.[35] Thereafter, a slower rate of decrease suggests maintenance of suppression and not treatment failure. Similarly, the decline in height velocity is most rapid in the first 18 months, and then growth should occur at a steady prepubertal rate.[35] It is important to remember that the process leading to accelerated bone maturation is put on pause during treatment and not reversed, so that when treatment is discontinued, rapid progression of bone maturation resumes. This is important in assessing changes in PAH.

Bone maturation needs to slow enough to compensate for the decreased height velocity, so that there is a net gain in height potential. Initially, PAH will improve rapidly, concurrent with the decrease in BA/CA. Most studies show continuous improvement in PAH throughout treatment. When very young children are treated, PAH may eventually stabilize, yet ongoing treatment is necessary to preserve height potential.[35] Recent studies suggest that a treatment duration of at least 24 months, if not 36 months, is necessary to optimize height outcome. It is also important to note that mid-parental height (MPH) influences height outcome, and GnRHa treatment rarely results in an adult height that exceeds it.[36]

Discontinuation of Treatment

Age, BA, height velocity, peers, MPH, and PAH all need to be considered in the timing of treatment cessation, and thus decisions on discontinuation of treatment need to be individualized. For a girl in whom the goal is menstrual suppression, grade in school and psychosocial adjustment are also important. To date, no studies have been able to predict when the onset of menstruation will occur following cessation of GnRHa treatment. The average time to menarche across studies is 18 months, but the range is 3 months to 3 years. This is crucial information for families, who need to be prepared for the unpredictability of HPG axis reactivation post-GnRHa treatment. However, several studies have suggested an inverse relationship between time to menarche and age at discontinuation of therapy.[37,38]

Neither a chronologic age nor a BA alone is an absolute criterion for stopping treatment. Studies that suggest so are based on a wide range of clinical scenarios. Not all patients included had truly rapidly progressing puberty and were likely having less benefit from treatment. Some patients with a BA greater than 12 years continue to have a significant increase in PAH, so treatment may be continued past this point if height is a concern.[31] Once CA and BA are equivalent, it is prudent to stop treatment for the sake of bone mineral density (BMD). BMD standard deviation score (SDS) decreases on GnRHa treatment, but because children with CPP have a BMD closer to normal for BA, post-treatment BMD is normal. Taken together, this implies not to treat past a BA = CA.

Outcomes

Height

Height outcomes in rapidly progressive CPP have improved over time as more children are treated earlier with less delay in onset of treatment[39] (**Table 2**). Most children reach an adult height consistent with genetic potential. There continue to be studies on optimizing height outcome through a careful evaluation of duration of treatment and timing of discontinuation of therapy.[31] A meta-analysis of controlled prospective studies showed that GnRHa therapy resulted in an increase in adult height compared with pretreatment height prediction of 0.63 SD score (95% CI 0.17–1.08).[36] It is important to note the range of height outcomes, as the average likely reflects a heterogeneous population, some of whom may not have been rigorously defined to have rapid CPP. In addition, the earlier studies included girls with a longer delay in the onset of treatment because GnRHas were newly available. Therefore, we highlight the importance of individualized decisions and assessments, as well as continued studies of adult height posttreatment with the newer GnRHas.

Reproductive function

Ovulatory function and menstrual cycles are normal once menses resume posttreatment.[4,40] Fertility and pregnancy outcomes are comparable to control populations[41] (**Table 3**). Since follow-up has extended only to women in their fourth decade of life, the timing of menopause is as yet unknown.[23] Further study is needed regarding the incidence of polycystic ovary syndrome (PCOS) in patients with a history of

Table 2
Height outcomes in different studies including study design and sample size

Author, Year of Publication (PMID)	Number of Girls	Years of GnRHa Treatment	Adult Height Achieved (cm)	Increase Above Predicted (cm)
Heger et al,[49] 1999 (10599723)	50	4.4 ± 2.1	160.6 ± 8.0	5.7
Antoniazzi et al, 2000 (10969920)	71	1.3–4.5	154.4 ± 5.6	2–7
Lazar et al, 2007 (17579199)	115	2.8–4.8	160.35 ± 5.05	5
Pasquino et al, 2008 (17940112)	87	4.2 ± 1.6	159.8 ± 5.3	5.1
Nabhan et al, 2009 (19554804)	26	3.6 ± 2.1	163 ± 7.6	4.5
Magiakou et al, 2010 (19897682)	33	2.75	158.5	6.95
Poomthavorn et al, 2011 (21501002)	47	3.4 ± 1.5	158.6 ± 5.2	4.7
Bertelloni et al, 2015 (26528763)	25	3.05 ± 0.9	158.25 ± 5.8	3
Lee et al, 2018 (30133462)	84	2.98 ± .73	160.1 ± 5	4
Trujillo et al,[31] 2021 (33856747)	38	3.9 ± 2.0	162.5 ± 7.4	5.3–7.3
Knific et al, 2022 (36531464)	48	~2	161.5 ± 7.5	−3.5
Cho et al,[27] 2023 (36690835)	188	3.21 ± 0.73	161.1 ± 4.8	4.72 ± 5

CPP, and whether treatment with GnRHas modifies this risk. Results from different studies are conflicting, and variations in patient populations and study methodology contribute to the challenge of deriving firm conclusions.[42,43]

BMI
There are conflicting studies regarding the impact of GnRHas on weight gain and body mass index (BMI). Although some have reported weight gain during treatment,[44,45] others have not reported any significant change in weight or BMI.[46,47] It is recommended to counsel patients regarding the pretreatment weight trajectory and importance of a healthy lifestyle, because height velocity slows once treatment is initiated. Women with a history of CPP have similar adult weight to the general population.[48]

Bone mineral density
BMD accrual is greatest during the pubertal years and children with CPP have higher BMD than age-matched peers. The rate of BMD accrual slows during treatment with GnRHas but resumes posttreatment and no long-term deficits in BMD have been reported in children with CPP.[49]

FUTURE DIRECTIONS

Discoveries in normal reproductive physiology and identification of the genetic basis for some cases of CPP lay the groundwork for innovative approaches to diagnosis, monitoring, and treatment. Future studies will likely explore the potential for targeted new treatments of CPP based on an understanding of the role of the kisspeptin system and the influence of the MKRN3 gene on the timing of puberty. An alternative approach to therapy that will likely become available even sooner is that of a GnRH antagonist, the pill form of which has been shown to have excellent efficacy and safety in men with prostate cancer and has been approved by the Food and Drug Administration (FDA) for this indication.[50] It is anticipated that clinical trials using this medication for the treatment of CPP in children will be initiated in the near future.

Table 3
Reproductive outcomes following gonadotropin-releasing hormone analog use for central precocious puberty

	Females		Males
Time to menarche	• Occurs 1–1.5 y after cessation of treatment on average but with wide individual variation (3 mo–3 y) • Inversely proportional to age and BA at cessation of treatment	Time to resumption of testicular enlargement	• Within 1 year following cessation of treatment
Ovulatory cycles	• Equal to that of controls without a history of CPP	Hormone concentrations (gonadotropins, testosterone, inhibin B)	• Equal to those of controls without a history of CPP
Time to conception	• Equal to that of the general population	Sperm count	• Equal to that of the general population
Need for ART	• No increased need for ART compared with the general population	Paternity rates	• Unknown
PCOS	• Some studies have reported ≥25% incidence of PCOS in women with a history of CPP, whereas others have found no increased risk. • Rates of PCOS have been reported to be higher in women with untreated vs treated CPP	Age of andropause	• Unknown
Age of menopause	• Unknown		

Abbreviation: ART, assisted reproductive technology.

CLINICS CARE POINTS

- Several available gonadotropin-releasing hormone analogs (GnRHas) have received regulatory approval for use in children with central precocious puberty (CPP), and the therapeutic armamentarium is expanding.
- GnRHas are largely safe and efficacious in the treatment of CPP.
- The primary goal of treatment in CPP is to preserve adult height.
- GnRHas are also used in CPP to minimize adverse psychosocial outcomes, but definitive support for this treatment indication is lacking.

DISCLOSURE

E. Eugster participates as site PI in sponsored clinical trials investigating new treatments for precocious puberty. K.O. Klein has been a consultant for several of the pharmaceutical companies that manufacture or market GnRHa.

REFERENCES

1. Apter D, Butzow TL, Laughlin GA, et al. Gonadotropin-releasing hormone pulse generator activity during pubertal transition in girls: pulsatile and diurnal patterns of circulating gonadotropins. J Clin Endocrinol Metab 1993;76(4):940–9.
2. Biro FM, Greenspan LC, Galvez MP, et al. Onset of breast development in a longitudinal cohort. Pediatrics 2013;132(6):1019–27.
3. Biro FM, Pajak A, Wolff MS, et al. Age of Menarche in a Longitudinal US Cohort. J Pediatr Adolesc Gynecol 2018;31(4):339–45.
4. Bangalore Krishna K, Fuqua JS, Rogol AD, et al. Use of gonadotropin-releasing hormone analogs in children: update by an international consortium. Horm Res Paediatr 2019;91(6):357–72.
5. Palmert MR, Malin HV, Boepple PA. Unsustained or slowly progressive puberty in young girls: initial presentation and long-term follow-up of 20 untreated patients. J Clin Endocrinol Metab 1999;84(2):415–23.
6. Biro FM, McMahon RP, Striegel-Moore R, et al. Impact of timing of pubertal maturation on growth in black and white female adolescents: The National Heart, Lung, and Blood Institute Growth and Health Study. J Pediatr 2001;138(5):636–43.
7. Franzini IA, Yamamoto FM, Bolfi F, et al. GnRH analog is ineffective in increasing adult height in girls with puberty onset after 7 years of age: a systematic review and meta-analysis. Eur J Endocrinol 2018;179(6):381–90.
8. Mendle J, Ryan RM, McKone KMP. Age at menarche, depression, and antisocial behavior in adulthood. Pediatrics 2018;141(1).
9. Mendle J, Ryan RM, McKone KMP. Early menarche and internalizing and externalizing in adulthood: explaining the persistence of effects. J Adolesc Health 2019;65(5):599–606.
10. Belchetz PE, Plant TM, Nakai Y, et al. Hypophysial responses to continuous and intermittent delivery of hypopthalamic gonadotropin-releasing hormone. Science 1978;202(4368):631–3.
11. Eugster EA, Clarke W, Kletter GB, et al. Efficacy and safety of histrelin subdermal implant in children with central precocious puberty: a multicenter trial. JClinEndocrinolMetab 2007;92(5):1697–704.
12. Lewis KA, Goldyn AK, West KW, et al. A single histrelin implant is effective for 2 years for treatment of central precocious puberty. J Pediatr 2013;163(4):1214–6.
13. Ray LA, Eckert GJ, Eugster EA. Long-term experience with the use of a single histrelin implant beyond one year in patients with central precocious puberty. J Pediatr Endocrinol Metab 2023;36(3):309–12.
14. Lee PA, Klein K, Mauras N, et al. 36-month treatment experience of two doses of leuprolide acetate 3-month depot for children with central precocious puberty. JClinEndocrinolMetab 2014;99(9):3153–9.
15. Fuqua JS. Treatment and outcomes of precocious puberty: an update. J Clin Endocrinol Metab 2013;98(6):2198–207.
16. Durand A, Tauber M, Patel B, et al. Meta-Analysis of Paediatric Patients with Central Precocious Puberty Treated with Intramuscular Triptorelin 11.25 mg 3-Month Prolonged-Release Formulation. Horm Res Paediatr 2017;87(4):224–32.

17. Klein K, Yang J, Aisenberg J, et al. Efficacy and safety of triptorelin 6-month formulation in patients with central precocious puberty. J Pediatr Endocrinol Metab 2016;29(11):1241–8.

18. Klein KO, Freire A, Gryngarten MG, et al. Phase 3 trial of a small-volume subcutaneous 6-month duration leuprolide acetate treatment for central precocious puberty. J Clin Endocrinol Metab 2020;105(10):e3660–71.

19. Klein KO, Mauras N, Nayak S, et al. Efficacy and safety of leuprolide acetate 6-month depot for the treatment of central precocious puberty: a phase 3 study. J Endocr Soc 2023;7(7):bvad071.

20. Aguirre RS, Eugster EA. Central precocious puberty: From genetics to treatment. Best Pract Res Clin Endocrinol Metabol 2018;32(4):343–54.

21. Chen M, Eugster EA. Central Precocious Puberty: Update on Diagnosis and Treatment. Pediatr Drugs 2015;17(4):273–81.

22. Miller BS, Shukla AR. Sterile abscess formation in response to two separate branded long-acting gonadotropin-releasing hormone agonists. Clin Therapeut 2010;32(10):1749–51.

23. Cantas-Orsdemir S, Eugster EA. Update on central precocious puberty: from etiologies to outcomes. Expert Rev Endocrino 2019;14(2):123–30.

24. De Sanctis V, Soliman AT, Di Maio S, et al. Long-term effects and significant Adverse Drug Reactions (ADRs) associated with the use of Gonadotropin-Releasing Hormone analogs (GnRHa) for central precocious puberty: a brief review of literature. Acta Biomed 2019;90(3):345–59.

25. Gohil A, Eugster EA. Gonadotropin-releasing hormone analogs for treatment of central precocious puberty in children younger than 2 years of age. J Pediatr Urol 2022;244:215–8.

26. Eugster EA. Treatment of central precocious puberty. J Endocr Soc 2019;3(5):965–72.

27. Cho AY, Shim YS, Lee HS, et al. Effect of gonadotropin-releasing hormone agonist monotherapy and combination therapy with growth hormone on final adult height in girls with central precocious puberty. Sci Rep 2023;13(1):1264.

28. Zhu S, Long L, Hu Y, et al. GnRHa/stanozolol combined therapy maintains normal bone growth in central precocious puberty. Front Endocrinol 2021;12:678797.

29. Vottero A, Pedori S, Verna M, et al. Final height in girls with central idiopathic precocious puberty treated with gonadotropin-releasing hormone analog and oxandrolone. J Clin Endocrinol Metab 2006;91(4):1284–7.

30. Liu S, Liu Q, Cheng X, et al. Effects and safety of combination therapy with gonadotropin-releasing hormone analogue and growth hormone in girls with idiopathic central precocious puberty: a meta-analysis. J Endocrinol Invest 2016;39(10):1167–78.

31. Vargas Trujillo M, Dragnic S, Aldridge P, et al. Importance of individualizing treatment decisions in girls with central precocious puberty when initiating treatment after age 7 years or continuing beyond a chronological age of 10 years or a bone age of 12 years. J Pediatr Endocrinol Metab 2021;34(6):733–9.

32. Neely EK, Lee PA, Bloch CA, et al. Leuprolide acetate 1-month depot for central precocious puberty: hormonal suppression and recovery. Int J Pediatr Endocrinol 2010;2010:398639.

33. Neely EK, Silverman LA, Geffner ME, et al. Random unstimulated pediatric luteinizing hormone levels are not reliable in the assessment of pubertal suppression during histrelin implant therapy. Int J Pediatr Endocrinol 2013;2013(1):20.

34. Lewis KA, Eugster EA. Random luteinizing hormone often remains pubertal in children treated with the histrelin implant for central precocious puberty. J Pediatr 2013;162(3):562–5.

35. Trujillo MV, Lee PA, Reifschneider K, et al. Using change in predicted adult height during GnRH agonist treatment for individualized treatment decisions in girls with central precocious puberty. J Pediatr Endocrinol Metab 2023;36(3):299–308.

36. Li P, Li Y, Yang CL. Gonadotropin releasing hormone agonist treatment to increase final stature in children with precocious puberty: a meta-analysis. Medicine (Baltim) 2014;93(27):e260.

37. Fisher MM, Lemay D, Eugster EA. Resumption of puberty in girls and boys following removal of the histrelin implant. J Pediatr 2014;164(4):912–916 e1.

38. Thornton P, Silverman LA, Geffner ME, et al. Review of outcomes after cessation of gonadotropin-releasing hormone agonist treatment of girls with precocious puberty. Pediatr Endocrinol Rev 2014;11(3):306–17.

39. Eugster EA. Treatment of Central Precocious Puberty. Journal of the Endocrine Society 2019;3(5):965–72.

40. Carel JC, Eugster EA, Rogol A, et al. Consensus statement on the use of gonadotropin-releasing hormone analogs in children. Pediatrics 2009;123(4):e752–62.

41. Guaraldi F, Beccuti G, Gori D, et al. Management of endocrine disease: Long-term outcomes of the treatment of central precocious puberty. Eur J Endocrinol 2016;174(3):R79–87.

42. Azziz R, Woods KS, Reyna R, et al. The prevalence and features of the polycystic ovary syndrome in an unselected population. J Clin Endocrinol Metab 2004;89(6):2745–9.

43. Rosenfield RL. Clinical review: Identifying children at risk for polycystic ovary syndrome. J Clin Endocrinol Metab 2007;92(3):787–96.

44. Traggiai C, Perucchin PP, Zerbini K, et al. Outcome after depot gonadotrophin-releasing hormone agonist treatment for central precocious puberty: effects on body mass index and final height. Eur J Endocrinol 2005;153(3):463–4.

45. Wolters B, Lass N, Reinehr T. Treatment with gonadotropin-releasing hormone analogues: different impact on body weight in normal-weight and overweight children. Horm Res Paediatr 2012;78(5–6):304–11.

46. Palmert MR, Mansfield MJ, Crowley WF, et al. Is obesity an outcome of gonadotropin-releasing hormone agonist administration? Analysis of growth and body composition in 110 patients with central precocious puberty. J Clin Endocrinol Metab 1999;84(12):4480–8.

47. Boot AM, De Muinck Keizer-Schrama S, Pols HA, et al. Bone mineral density and body composition before and during treatment with gonadotropin-releasing hormone agonist in children with central precocious and early puberty. J Clin Endocrinol Metab 1998;83(2):370–3.

48. Lazar L, Lebenthal Y, Yackobovitch-Gavan M, et al. Treated and untreated women with idiopathic precocious puberty: BMI evolution, metabolic outcome, and general health between third and fifth decades. J Clin Endocrinol Metab 2015;100(4):1445–51.

49. Heger S, Partsch CJ, Sippell WG. Long-term outcome after depot gonadotropin-releasing hormone agonist treatment of central precocious puberty: final height, body proportions, body composition, bone mineral density, and reproductive function. J Clin Endocrinol Metab 1999;84(12):4583–90.

50. Shore ND, Saad F, Cookson MS, et al, HERO Study Investigators. Oral relugolix for androgen-deprivation therapy in advanced prostate cancer. N Engl J Med 2020;382(23):2187–96.

Diagnosis, Treatment, and Outcomes of Males with Central Precocious Puberty

Renée Robilliard, DO[a,b], Peter A. Lee, MD, PhD[c],*,
Lisa Swartz Topor, MD, MMSc[a,b]

KEYWORDS

- Precocious puberty • Gonadotropin-releasing hormone analogue • Short stature

KEY POINTS

- Central precocious puberty (CPP) is defined by onset of centrally activated puberty in boys prior to the age of 9 year old.
- All male patients who have biochemical CPP are recommended to have a brain MRI to evaluate the hypothalamic-pituitary region for lesions. In boys with CPP, 36% to 74% will have a detectable central nervous system lesion.
- Without treatment to halt pubertal progression, some boys with CPP will have premature closure of growth plates and reduced adult height compared to genetic potential.
- Gonadotropin-releasing hormone (GnRH) agonist treatment can halt CPP. These medications can be delivered in intramuscular, subdermal, subcutaneous, or intranasal formulations or implants. Treatment slows growth velocity and pubertal progression and increases predicted adult height during therapy, though long-term data describing boys treated for CPP are lacking.

INTRODUCTION

The typical timing of male puberty begins between 9 and 14 years old, at an average age of 11.6 ± 0.9 years.[1] Luteinizing hormone (LH), measured via an ultrasensitive assay, acts as a surrogate marker for gonadotropin-releasing hormone (GnRH) in serum laboratory studies. Central precocious puberty (CPP) is caused by a release of inhibition on pulsatile GnRH secretion.[2] Onset of puberty in boys is documented by a random LH level ≥ 0.3 IU/L or a peak LH > 5 IU/L after GnRH agonist (GnRHa) stimulation testing (subcutaneous leuprolide, 10 ug/kg)[3] with an increase in testicular

Funding/support: No specific funding/support.
[a] Division of Pediatric Endocrinology and Diabetes, Hasbro Children's Hospital, Providence, RI, USA; [b] Warren Alpert Medical School of Brown University, Providence, RI, USA; [c] Division of Pediatric Endocrinology, Department of Pediatrics, Penn State College of Medicine, Hershey, PA, USA
* Corresponding author. 12 Briarcrest Square, Hershey, PA 17033.
E-mail address: plee@psu.edu

Endocrinol Metab Clin N Am 53 (2024) 239–250
https://doi.org/10.1016/j.ecl.2024.01.005   **endo.theclinics.com**
0889-8529/24/© 2024 Elsevier Inc. All rights reserved.

volume >3 mL. Pulsatile LH stimulates Leydig cells to produce testosterone. These findings prior to the age of 9 year old are consistent with CPP .[2]

INCIDENCE AND SECULAR TRENDS

The estimated incidence of CPP ranges from 0.01 to 2/10,000 children in boys, which is less frequent than in girls (CPP rates of 0.1–26.3/10,000).[4] Unlike female puberty, which has trended to become earlier over the past 3 decades, studies in boys in different regions have had conflicting findings. While Korean and Turkish studies suggest increasing rates of CPP in boys,[4] a US study from 2001 to 2010 did not show a change in frequency of CPP in males.[5] Possible causes for the discordance between timing of onset may be definitions, visual inspection versus physical examination, laboratory verification of LH levels, and type of study performed.[6] This is an area that requires further exploration.

UNDERLYING CAUSES

Genetics, adiposity, nutritional status, environmental and chemical exposures, and chronic illnesses can impact pubertal timing in girls. However, there is limited evidence to link these to the development of CPP in males.[7] A Danish study (846 boys) examined the relationship between timing of puberty in parents and sons and found early pubertal timing of parents was associated with earlier pubertal onset in sons compared to boys with average or late maturing parents.[6] A 2022 multi-center cohort study examined the transition into puberty in adolescents born between 2003 to 2011 (68,571 boys), using age at transition from Tanner stage 1 to Tanner stage 2+ as a primary outcome.[8] Boys with overweight or obese body mass index (BMI) had earlier gonadarche compared with boys with BMI in the normal range. Underweight boys had a decreased likelihood of earlier gonadarche.[8] These findings contrast with the outcomes of prior studies, which have shown an inverse relationship between elevated BMI z-scores and age of onset of pubertal development.[9] A 2016 study found an association between earlier puberty in overweight boys and later pubertal onset in obese White non-Hispanic adolescent boys.[10]

Environmental pollutants can act as endocrine disrupting chemicals. Compounds investigated for a role in impacting pubertal timing include phthalates, bisphenol A, polychlorinated biphenyls (PCBs), perfluorooctanesulfonic acid (PFOS), and organochlorine pesticides.[11] Evidence that links exposure to alterations in timing in male puberty is limited. Some studies have shown delayed male puberty in PCB-exposed and PFOS-exposed boys,[11] and further research is needed in this area.

Primary underlying causes of CPP in males are predominantly due to central nervous system (CNS) lesions and genetic conditions, while idiopathic causes account for 10% of cases.[12] CPP is more often due to an underlying cause in males, whereas idiopathic CPP is the most common finding in girls.[4] CNS lesions associated with CPP include hypothalamic hamartomas, germ cell tumors, glial cell tumors, craniopharyngioma, and pinealomas, though any CNS lesion can be associated with CPP. Congenital brain defects such as midline anomalies, cranial irradiation, history of infection, or trauma can also be associated with CPP. Underlying genetic conditions, including neurofibromatosis-1 and tuberous sclerosis, can be risk factors for developing CPP.[2,4] (**Table 1**).

Genetic Mutations

Genetic mutations have been identified as causes of familial CPP. The most common genetic cause of CPP is loss of function mutations of the Makorin ring finger protein-3 gene (*MKRN3*). Due to the maternal imprinting inheritance pattern, CPP only occurs if

Table 1
Underlying causes of male central precocious puberty[2,4]

Category	Condition	Comments
Central nervous system Lesions	Hypothalamic hamartoma Glial cell tumors Germ cell tumors Craniopharyngioma Pinealoma	
Congenital Brain Defects	Subarachnoid cyst Arachnoidocele Rathke cleft cyst	
Congenital Midline Anomalies	Hydrocephalus Meningomyelocele Optic nerve hypoplasia	
Non-Organic Causes	Cranial irradiation Previous meningoencephalitis Head trauma Perinatal insult	
Underlying condition	Neurofibromatosis, type 1 Tuberous sclerosis Untreated peripheral precocious puberty (CAH, exogenous testosterone exposure)	Activation of CP due to sex steroid exposure, known as secondary CPP
	Van Wyk–Grumbach syndrome	Longstanding untreated hypothyroidism, possibly caused by elevated TRH stimulating follicle stimulating hormone(FSH)/ Luteinizing hormone (LH) secretion
	Sturge–Weber syndrome Williams–Beuren syndrome Temple syndrome RASopathies	
Genetic Mutations	*KISS1* *KISS1R*	Gain of function mutation Gain of function mutation in the KISS1 receptor gene
	LIN28B *DLK1* *MKRN3* Chromosomal microdeletion (1p36, 9p)	Mechanism unknown Gain of function mutation Gain of function mutation
Idiopathic/Other	Associated with being adopted from abroad Ectopic neurohypophysis	

Abbreviations: CAH, congenital adrenal hyperplasia; CP, central puberty; TRH, thyrotropin-releasing hormone.

the mutated allele is inherited from the father. In mouse models, the function of *MKRN3* is primarily to inhibit pubertal initiation. One meta-analysis described *MKRN3* defects in 13 boys.[13] The boys experiencing CPP associated with a *MKRN3* defect had later onset of puberty compared to boys experiencing CPP without a *MKRN3* defect (8.2 vs 7 years, respectively).[14] The gene delta-like non-canonical notch ligand-1 (*DLK1*) is a paternally expressed transmembrane protein present in a variety of embryonic tissues. Defects in this gene are associated with higher risk of obesity, diabetes mellitus, and CPP.[15] In 2022, the first male patient with CPP due to a *DLK1* gene mutation was identified. His sister and father were also affected.[16] Mutations in genes associated with kisspeptin (*KISS1*) or its receptor (*KISS1R*) also cause CPP. Kisspeptin neurons are involved in pulsatile GnRH release, leading to onset of central puberty.[17] A heterozygous mutation (p.P74S) in *KISS1* was identified in a boy with sporadic CPP at age 12 months.[18]

Among the less common gene mutations associated with CPP, only a mutation in *NOTCH1* has been associated with a case of male CPP, and the rest have only been described in females.[19]

CLINICAL EVALUATION AND DIAGNOSIS

Boys with CPP typically have symmetric, pubertal sized (>3 cc) testes on examination. The presence of pubertal symptoms with pre-pubertal testes (volume $\leq$ 3 cc) indicates that androgens are being produced elsewhere, as is seen with premature adrenarche (a benign variant) or are from an adrenal or exogenous source (examples include congenital adrenal hyperplasia [CAH], adrenal tumors, and exogenous testosterone exposure). Asymmetric testicular volumes are not consistent with stimulation by circulating gonadotropins in CPP, and may indicate a peripheral source of androgens such as a testicular tumor.[7] Asymmetry may also result from earlier testicular damage or correction of cryptorchidism after infancy.

After determining that a male patient less than 9 year old has symmetrically enlarged (>3 cc) testes, the next step in evaluation is measurement of serum gonadotropins (follicle stimulating hormone[FSH]/luteinizing hormone [LH]) and total testosterone levels, which are typically elevated. Serum gonadotropin levels monitored by ultrasensitive assays are preferred and ideally obtained in the morning due to the pulsatile release and higher amplitude of gonadotropin action in the early morning during the initial stages of puberty.[4,12] Human chorionic gonadotropin (hCG) is also measured to rule out pathologic elevation which can occur in the setting of certain tumors.

If, despite low or pre-pubertal gonadotropin levels, there remains a high level of clinical suspicion for CPP, a GnRH stimulation test is the next step in evaluation, as described in (see Kanthi Bangalore Krishna and Lawrence A. Silverman's article, "Diagnosis of Central Precocious Puberty," in this issue). Measurement of pubertal levels of LH after GnRH stimulation indicates that endogenous GnRH exposure has "primed" the pituitary gonadotrophs.[20] The laboratory findings most typical in CPP include pubertal unstimulated gonadotropin levels or elevated gonadotropins after GnRH stimulation testing, undetectable serum hCG, and elevated serum testosterone levels.

Once CPP is identified, the next step is to evaluate if there is an underlying cause (see **Table 1**) and to assess the tempo of pubertal progression. A bone age (BA) significantly advanced for chronologic age indicates greater exposure to sex steroids. If the BA is consistent with chronologic age, then it is less likely that the patient has had significant exposure to high concentrations of sex steroids.[2]

All male patients who have biochemical CPP require a brain MRI with contrast to evaluate the hypothalamic-pituitary region for lesions. In contrast to girls, who are likely to have idiopathic CPP, boys are more likely (36%–74% in various studies) to have a CNS lesion associated with CPP.[4,5]

TREATMENT

Decisions surrounding treatment initiation should consider underlying etiology, family history, height prediction, and tempo of pubertal progression. In patients with a strong family history of onset within the early range, but not central precocious puberty, with rapid advancement of physical development, this variation of normal may require treatment. In the absence of rapid pubertal progression or psychosocial distress, a 3-to-6-month period of observation can be considered prior to initiation of treatment.[20] Goals of treatment in males are (1) halt further development of secondary sexual characteristics, (2) prevent psychological disturbance, and (3) preserve final adult height (FAH).[20,21] However, criteria to identify patients who require treatment have not been established. Overall, the strongest indications for treatment are among younger patients, in those with BA advancement of more than 2 years beyond chronologic age, and in those with predicted adult height less than 165 cm or greater than 5 cm below mid-parental height.[20–22]

GnRHa are used to halt pubertal progression in boys with CPP through tonic GnRH action at the receptor, overriding the endogenous pulsatile release pattern that stimulates gonadotropins. The consistent presence of GnRH transiently leads to stimulation of GnRH receptors, followed by a downregulation of GnRH receptors on the pituitary. This downregulation causes decreased sensitivity to GnRH and reduction in release of gonadotropins, which halts stimulation of the testes to produce testosterone. Available GnRHa formulations are described in **Table 2**. Specific guidelines about discontinuation of GnRHa in boys do not currently exist, but typically therapy is continued until approximately age 12 years.[20,21]

Clinical evaluation is used to assess response to pubertal suppression with GnRHa and should be completed every 3 to 6 months with measurement of growth velocity (GV) and Tanner staging. BA can be monitored periodically, with an expectation that the rate of BA advancement slows by a year after beginning GnRHa therapy.[20] To assess biochemical efficacy, serum LH levels can be measured prior to a GnRHa dose, with a goal of LH in the pre-pubertal range. In patients with a histrelin implant, LH levels may not be suppressed in approximately 60% of cases, so clinical assessment is the most effective way to assess efficacy of treatment.[20,23]

When GnRHa therapy is discontinued, the hypothalamic–pituitary–gonadal (HPG) axis typically shows signs of reactivation well before 12 months. The most common short-term side effect associated with leuprolide is sterile abscess at injection sites.[20,21]

Various formulations of GnRHa treatment for CPP have been evaluated. Study cohorts mainly include girls due to their higher frequency of CPP. As a result, there is

Table 2
Currently available formulations of gonadotropin-releasing hormone analogs[27,28]

Drug Name	Route of Administration	Frequency of Administration
Leuprolide acetate depot	IM, SQ injection	1-mo, 3-mo, or 6-mo formulations
Histrelin	Subdermal implant	1–2 y
Triptorelin	IM injection	1-mo, 3-mo, or 6-mo formulations
Nafarelin acetate (rarely used)	Intranasal	Every 12 h
Leuprolide acetate (rarely used)	Subcutaneous injection	Daily

limited information about these medications in male patients, and specific outcomes in the male patients were not reported in the studies. A study on the 3-month formulation of triptorelin (11.25 mg) demonstrated adequate LH suppression at 3, 6, and 12 months after treatment initiation in 4 out of 5 boys.[24] Two studies of the 3-month formulations of leuprolide acetate (11.25 mg, 30 mg) included 7 and 8 boys, respectively, and a study utilizing the 6-month (45 mg) formulation included 2 boys.[25–27] Both 3-month formulations (11.25 and 30 mg) and the 6-month (45 mg) formulation preparations were effective at suppressing pubertal progression after 6 months of use.[25–27] A study of the 6-month formulation of triptorelin, which included 9 boys, reported effective suppression of gonadotropins and improved predicted adult height (PAH) during the treatment course.[28]

OUTCOMES OF TREATED AND UNTREATED CENTRAL PRECOCIOUS PUBERTY IN MALES

Due to the rare incidence of idiopathic CPP in boys, limited data regarding treatment outcomes in males are available. **Table 3** summarizes previous unreported outcome data for 3 men now in their 40s. For the 2 men who did not have a pre-existing condition, their outcome was excellent, including social interactions, work, family relationships, and fertility, while treatment was begun so late that they had compromised adult heights. Published outcome information is included in the following paragraphs according to topics.

Growth Velocity and Final Adult Height

Without treatment to halt pubertal progression, some boys with CPP will have reduced adult height, up to 3 standard deviations below normal values for matched peers.[22] An analysis of adult height in 9 boys (age 6.0 ± 1.8 years at therapy initiation) with CPP treated with GnRHa therapy (duration 5.6 ± 2.4 years) found final adult height (FAH) to be significantly higher than the initial predicted adult height (PAH) at time of evaluation, and within range for mid parental height. The outcomes did not differ based upon type or duration of GnRH analog used or underlying cause of CPP.[29] A study of 23 boys treated for CPP with GnRHa therapy showed improved PAH after 12 months of therapy compared to baseline predictions. They also found that after 12 months of therapy, GV decreased from baseline, suggesting a decline in growth acceleration, with the expectation that growth plate maturation would also slow and allow more time for linear growth.[30] FAH was not reported in this study. Multiple other studies have showed slowed GV during GnRHa treatment and increased PAH during therapy.[31–33] A retrospective study of 18 boys with CPP who were evaluated prior to GnRHa treatment, 1 year into GnRH treatment, and once FAH was reached showed that FAH was consistent with and slightly greater than mid-parental height (172.0 ± 4.8 cm vs 171.4 ± 4.0 cm respectively). These results support improved growth potential with GnRHa treatment.[33,34] Studies have shown that growth after cessation of GnRHa therapy is correlated with BA at time of discontinuation of treatment, and that discontinuation of treatment at a BA close to peak height velocity may be most beneficial to improve FAH.[22]

Augmentation of Growth in Addition to Gonadotropin-Releasing Hormone Agonist Therapy

Aromatase inhibitors (AI) have been explored as part of growth-promoting treatment for boys with short stature (idiopathic short stature, familial male-limited precocious puberty), but publications about AI use in boys with CPP are limited to case

Table 3
Previously unpublished long-term follow-up of 3 patients

		Patient 1	Patient 2	Patient 3
Age (years)	Current	47	47	41
	At diagnosis	9.4	10.2	9.8
	At therapy onset	9.5	10.7	10.8
	At end of therapy	12.4	13.3	14.5
Gonadotropin-releasing hormone agonist (GnRHa)	Daily Aqueous/1 mo. Depot	Aqueous	Aqueous	Depot
	Duration	3.0	2.8	3.7
Height (cm)	At diagnosis	145.6	148.9	156.0
	At onset of therapy	147.2	153.9	160.3
	At end of therapy	163.6	168.3	178.3
	Target height range	1.57–1.83	Adopted	1.63–1.80
	Predicted adult height (AH) onset of therapy	167.5	179.9	175.0
	PAH end of therapy	170.4	176.4	180.1
	Growth post-Rx	8.5	2.8	1.3
	Adult height	172.1	171.1	179.6
Skeletal age	At onset of therapy	13.25	14.25	13.0
	At end of therapy	13.5	14.5	17.0
Academic achievement		BA with honors, MA-full scholarship	Poor attention deficit hyperactivity disorder, Intellectual disability	College
Physical fitness		Excellent	Poor	Good
Employment		Corporate VP	Restaurant (25 y)	IT (25y)
Partner pregnancy		X3, 1–3 mo attempting	NA	Yes, first month attempting
Children	Sex and Age	Male 17 y Female 13 y Male 9 y	NA	Female 9 y
	Medical conditions	Healthy, normal puberty	NA	None
Significant medical conditions		None	Obesity post-treatment	None
Perception of GnRHa therapy benefit		Hoped to be even taller	"Probably helped"	Hoped to be even taller
Perception of impact of central precocious puberty (CPP)		Assumed that he would be taller because of height during childhood	Still unaware of the fact that his puberty was early	Bullied after being placed with older teens

(continued on next page)

Table 3 (continued)			
	Patient 1	Patient 2	Patient 3
Comments	Remarkably well-adjusted adult. Accepts adult height. Commendable family, work, and social life.	Therapy stopped because of slow growth. Prostate massage swab showed living sperm	Wonders if erectile dysfunction started earlier due to CPP

reports.[35,36] A male with CPP with prior attempted surgery for a hamartoma not treated with GnRHa was treated with anastrozole 1 mg daily for 3 years and the patient had a gain of 6 cm compared to the initial PAH.[37]

Few studies have examined the use of growth hormone (GH) in conjunction with GnRHa therapy in children with CPP.[38] One study of 14 children (10 girls, 4 boys) who had a decline in GV to less than the 25th percentile during treatment for CPP and had no improvement in PAH were treated with GH (0.3 mg/kg/week) for 2 to 3 years. Outcomes in boys showed no significant change in GV throughout treatment but did show improvement in PAH in the first year after combined treatment. However, the change in PAH was not statistically significant, and FAH had not been achieved at the time of publication.[31,38]

Body Mass Index and Cardiovascular Effects

A retrospective study of children previously treated with GnRHa for CPP showed no significant difference in BMI from the start to end of therapy or at a time measured later when they were near FAH.[39] There was no difference in glucose or lipid values between treated patients and controls, implying GnRHa therapy had minimal effects.[39] A Portuguese study (8 boys with CPP) showed that boys were heavier than girls prior to treatment and did not have an increase in BMI z-score during treatment. Both sexes had a decreased BMI z-score from baseline to a year after ending GnRHa therapy.[40] A study of the histrelin implant found a decrease in BMI percentiles in all patients (29 girls, 2 boys) at 24 months of treatment compared to baseline, though outcomes over a longer duration were not reported.[23]

Fertility Outcomes

A limited number of studies examined long-term gonadal function in males with CPP after GnRHa treatment and reported normal gonadal function and no alteration in serum testosterone levels or semen analyses compared to males with normal pubertal timing.[29,41] One study of 14 patients (7 males) with CPP due to hypothalamic hamartoma found that at adulthood all subjects had normal gonadal function; 3 males had fathered children.[42]

Bone Mineral Density

Bone mineral mass increases throughout childhood and during puberty. Compared to pre-pubertal girls, pre-pubertal boys have slightly higher total body bone mineral content.[43] One longitudinal study of children treated with GnRHa therapy for CPP (2 boys) showed that when corrected for BA, children had normal bone mineral density (BMD) before, during, and after treatment.[44] One Italian study of 9 males treated with GnRHa therapy found that after therapy (mean age 16.7 ± 1.5 years), BMD values were within normal range and comparable to men with average onset of pubertal timing.[29]

Psychosocial Outcomes

There are limited studies assessing the psychosocial functioning of males with treated or untreated CPP. One study of caregivers of 3491 children (50.8% boys) reported that in boys with signs of puberty by age 8 to 9, there was worse psychosocial adjustment from early childhood through adolescence and increased behavioral difficulties.[45] A cross-sectional study of caregivers of patients with CPP (21 boys, 121 girls) found that children with CPP have poorer psychosocial health and emotional functioning compared to peers without CPP. Outcomes did not differ among children with CPP who had or had not undergone treatment. Results were not reported by gender.[46]

SUMMARY

CPP in males is rare, and long-term outcome studies on males with CPP are lacking. Males with CPP are more likely to have an underlying CNS cause, and therefore all boys with CPP require evaluation with brain MRI. While treatment of male CPP with GnRHa therapy leads to slowed growth velocity and increased predicted adult height, further studies need to be conducted to examine the impact of GnRHa treatment with respect to FAH, BMI, future fertility, and psychosocial outcomes.

CLINICS CARE POINTS

- The first sign of puberty in males is testicular growth; volume greater than 3 mL or longitudinal axis greater than 2.5 cm is indicative of growth.
- Central precocious puberty [early resurgence of the hypothalamic-pituitary-testicular (HPT) axis] is less common among males than females, although it is more likely to have an underlying pathologic cause. Hence, imaging studies of the CNS are done more frequently.
- GnRH analogs are the treatment of choice to halt pubertal development in males, and monitoring of therapy is simpler than among females, since suppressed testosterone levels are indicative of axis suppression.
- Limited outcome data indicate that therapy
  - preserves or reclaims growth potential depending upon degree of advancement of bone age at onset of therapy.
  - The HPT axis is active within months of stopping therapy.
- Available long-term outcome data indicate that quality of life (social, sexual, work, fertility) is normal among males after CPP and GnRHa therapy.

DISCLOSURE

The authors have no conflicts of interest to disclose.

REFERENCES

1. Marshall WA, Tanner JM. Variations in the pattern of pubertal changes in boys. Arch Dis Child 1970;45(239):13–23.
2. Carel JC, Leger J. Clinical practice. Precocious puberty. N Engl J Med 2008; 358(22):2366–77.
3. Neely EK, Wilson DM, Lee PA, et al. Spontaneous serum gonadotropin concentrations in the evaluation of precocious puberty. J Pediatr 1995;127:47–52.
4. Mucaria C, Tyutyusheva N, Baroncelli GI, et al. Central Precocious Puberty in Boys and Girls: Similarities and Differences. Sexes 2021;2(1):119–31.

5. Topor LS, Bowerman K, Machan JT, et al. Central precocious puberty in Boston boys: A 10-year single center experience. PLoS One 2018;13(6):e0199019.
6. Fuqua JS. Treatment and Outcomes of Precocious Puberty: An Update. J Clin Endocrinol Metab 2013;98(6):2198–207.
7. Chen M, Eugster EA. Central Precocious Puberty: Update on Diagnosis and Treatment. Paediatr Drugs 2015;17(4):273–81.
8. Aghaee S, Deardorff J, Quesenberry CP, et al. Associations Between Childhood Obesity and Pubertal Timing Stratified by Sex and Race/Ethnicity. Am J Epidemiol 2022;191(12):2026–36.
9. Busch AS, Hollis B, Day FR, et al. Voice break in boys-temporal relations with other pubertal milestones and likely causal effects of BMI. Hum Reprod 2019; 34(8):1514–22.
10. Lee JM, Wasserman R, Kaciroti N, et al. Timing of Puberty in Overweight Versus Obese Boys. Pediatrics 2016;137(2):e20150164.
11. Vested A, Giwercman A, Bonde JP, et al. Persistent organic pollutants and male reproductive health. Asian J Androl 2014;16(1):71–80.
12. Chan YM, Fenoglio-Simeone KA, Paraschos S, et al. Central precocious puberty due to hypothalamic hamartomas correlates with anatomic features but not with expression of GnRH, TGFalpha, or KISS1. Horm Res Paediatr 2010;73(5):312–9.
13. Valadares LP, Meireles CG, De Toledo IP, et al. *MKRN3* Mutations in Central Precocious Puberty: A Systematic Review and Meta-Analysis. J Endocr Soc 2019; 3(5):979–95.
14. Bessa DS, Macedo DB, Brito VN, et al. High Frequency of MKRN3 Mutations in Male Central Precocious Puberty Previously Classified as Idiopathic. Neuroendocrinology 2017;105(1):17–25.
15. Pittaway JFH, Lipsos C, Katia Marinie. The role of delta-like non-canonical Notch ligand 1 (DLK1) in cancer. Endocr Relat Cancer 2021;28(12):R271–87.
16. Palumbo S, Cirillo G, Sanchez G, et al. A new DLK1 defect in a family with idiopathic central precocious puberty: elucidation of the male phenotype. J Endocrinol Invest 2023;46(6):1233–40.
17. Tng EL. Kisspeptin signalling and its roles in humans. Singapore Med J 2015; 56(12):649–56.
18. Silveira LG, Noel SD, Silveira-Neto AP, et al. Mutations of the KISS1 Gene in Disorders of Puberty. J Clin Endocrinol Metab 2010;95(5):2276–80.
19. Moise-Silverman J, Silverman LA. A review of the genetics and epigenetics of central precocious puberty. Front Endocrinol 2022;13:1029137.
20. Carel JC, Eugster EA, Rogol A, Ghizzoni L, et al. Consensus statement on the use of gonadotropin-releasing hormone analogs in children. Pediatrics 2009;123(4): e752–62.
21. Kaplowitz PB. Treatment of central precocious puberty. Curr Opin Endocrinol Diabetes Obes 2009;16(1):31–6.
22. Bertelloni S, Mul D. Treatment of central precocious puberty by GnRH analogs: long-term outcome in men. Asian J Androl 2008;10(4):525–34.
23. Rahhal S, Clarke WL, Kletter GB, et al. Results of a Second Year of Therapy with the 12-Month Histrelin Implant for the Treatment of Central Precocious Puberty. Int J Pediatr Endocrinol 2009. https://doi.org/10.1155/2009/812517. https://www.ncbi.nlm.nih.gov/pmc/articles/PMC2777002/.
24. Carel JC, Blumberg J, Seymour C, et al. Triptorelin 3-month CPP Study Group. Three-month sustained-release triptorelin (11.25 mg) in the treatment of central precocious puberty. Eur J Endocrinol 2006;154(1):119–24.

25. Klein KO, Freire A, Gryngarten MG, et al. Phase 3 Trial of a Small-volume Subcutaneous 6-Month Duration Leuprolide Acetate Treatment for Central Precocious Puberty. J Clin Endocrinol Metab 2020;105(10):e3660–71. Erratum in: J Clin Endocrinol Metab. 2021 Jun 16;106(7):e2842.

26. Lee PA, Klein K, Mauras N, et al. 36-month treatment experience of two doses of leuprolide acetate 3-month depot for children with central precocious puberty. J Clin Endocrinol Metab 2014;99(9):3153–9.

27. Lee PA, Klein K, Mauras N, et al. Efficacy and safety of leuprolide acetate 3-month depot 11.25 milligrams or 30 milligrams for the treatment of central precocious puberty. J Clin Endocrinol Metab 2012;97(5):1572–80.

28. Popovic J, Geffner ME, Rogol AD, et al. Gonadotropin-releasing hormone analog therapies for children with central precocious puberty in the United States. Front Pediatr 2022;10:968485.

29. Bertelloni S, Baroncelli GI, Ferdeghini M, et al. Final height, gonadal function and bone mineral density of adolescent males with central precocious puberty after therapy with gonadotropin-releasing hormone analogues. Eur J Pediatr 2000; 159(5):369–74.

30. Ni MM, Yang ST, Wu WW, et al. Benefits from the first year of GnRHa therapy in boys with idiopathic central precocious puberty when initiating treatment after age 9 years: findings from a real-world retrospective study. BMC Endocr Disord 2022;22(1):299.

31. Pasquino AM, Municchi G, Pucarelli I, et al. Combined treatment with gonadotropin-releasing hormone analog and growth hormone in central precocious puberty. J Clin Endocrinol Metab 1996;81(3):948–51.

32. Oostdijk W, Hümmelink R, Odink RJ, et al. Treatment of children with central precocious puberty by a slow-release gonadotropin-releasing hormone agonist. Eur J Pediatr 1990;149(5):308–13.

33. Shim YS, Lim KI, Lee HS, et al. Long-term outcomes after gonadotropin-releasing hormone agonist treatment in boys with central precocious puberty. PLoS One 2020;15(12):e0243212.

34. Cho AY, Ko SY, Lee JH, et al. Effects of gonadotropin-releasing hormone agonist treatment on final adult height in boys with idiopathic central precocious puberty. Ann Pediatr Endocrinol Metab 2021;26(4):259–65.

35. Mauras N, Ross J, Mericq V. Management of Growth Disorders in Puberty: GH, GnRHa, and Aromatase Inhibitors: A clinical review. Endocr Rev 2023;44:1–13.

36. Wit J. Should Skeletal Maturation Be Manipulated for Extra Height Gain? Front Endocrinol 2021;(12). https://doi.org/10.3389/fendo.2021.812196.

37. Faglia G, Arosio M, Porretti S. Delayed closure of epiphyseal cartilages induced by the aromatase inhibitor anastrozole. Would it help short children grow up? J Endocrinol Invest 2000;23(11):721–3.

38. Walvoor EC, Pescovitz OH. Combined Use of Growth Hormone and Gonadotropin-releasing Hormone Analogues in Precocious Puberty: Theoretic and Practical Considerations. Pediatrics 1999;104:1010–4.

39. Chiocca E, Dati E, Baroncelli G, et al. Body Mass Index and Body Composition in Adolescents Treated with Gonadotropin-Releasing Hormone Analogue Triptorelin Depot for Central Precocious Puberty: Data at Near Final Height. Neuroendocrinology 2009;89(4):441–7.

40. Leite AL, Galo E, Antunes A, et al. Do GnRH Agonists Really Increase Body Weight Gain? Evaluation of a Multicentric Portuguese Cohort of Patients With Central Precocious Puberty. Front Pediatr 2022 Mar 4;10:816635.

41. Tanaka T, Niimi H, Matsuo N, et al. Results of long-term follow-up after treatment of central precocious puberty with leuprorelin acetate: evaluation of effectiveness of treatment and recovery of gonadal function. The TAP-144-SR Japanese Study Group on Central Precocious Puberty. J Clin Endocrinol Metab 2005;90(3): 1371–6.

42. Ramos CO, Latronico AC, Cukier P, et al. Long-Term Outcomes of Patients with Central Precocious Puberty due to Hypothalamic Hamartoma after GnRHa Treatment: Anthropometric, Metabolic, and Reproductive Aspects. Neuroendocrinology 2018;106(3):203–10.

43. Gonc EN, Kandemir N. Body composition in sexual precocity. Curr Opin Endocrinol Diabetes Obes 2022;29(1):78–83.

44. Van Der Sluis IM, Boot AM, Krenning EP, et al. Longitudinal Follow-Up of Bone Density and Body Composition in Children with Precocious or Early Puberty before, during and after Cessation of GnRH Agonist Therapy. J Clin Endocrinol Metab 2002;87(2):506–512507.

45. Mensah FK, Bayer JK, Wake M, et al. Early Puberty and Childhood Social and Behavioral Adjustment. J Adoles Health 2013;53(1):118–24. ISSN 1054-139X.

46. Klein KO, Soliman AM, Grubb E, et al. A survey of care pathway and health-related quality of life impact for children with central precocious puberty. Curr Med Res Opin 2020;36(3):411–8.

Presentation and Care for Children with Peripheral Precocious Puberty

John S. Fuqua, MD*, Erica A. Eugster, MD

KEYWORDS

- Peripheral precocious puberty • McCune-Albright syndrome
- Familial male-limited precocious puberty • Congenital adrenal hyperplasia
- Testicular tumor • Ovarian tumor

KEY POINTS

- Peripheral precocious puberty (PPP) occurs when there is exposure to sex steroids that are not regulated by the central nervous system.
- Genetic causes of PPP include congenital adrenal hyperplasia, McCune-Albright syndrome, familial male-limited precocious puberty, and glucocorticoid resistance.
- Acquired causes of PPP include a variety of secretory gonadal tumors, human chorionic gonadotropin-secreting tumors, hypothyroidism, exogenous exposure, and ovarian cysts.

INTRODUCTION

Peripheral precocious puberty (PPP) refers to the early onset of sexual maturation that is independent of central nervous system (CNS) control. Causes of PPP include a variety of genetic disorders that increase sex hormone secretion. There are also many acquired causes of PPP, including tumors and exogenous hormone exposures **(Table 1)**. Treatment of PPP may include surgery, hormone blockade, or in some cases hormone replacement. This article will review both genetic and acquired causes of PPP, focusing on clinical presentation, diagnosis, and treatment.

DISTINGUISHING PERIPHERAL PRECOCIOUS PUBERTY FROM CENTRAL PRECOCIOUS PUBERTY

PPP must be distinguished from central precocious puberty (CPP). Clinically, this is more straightforward in boys due to the ability to palpate the testes. Causes of CPP lead to bilateral symmetric testicular growth because of the stimulatory effects of

Division of Pediatric Endocrinology, Indiana University School of Medicine, 705 Riley Hospital Drive, Room 5960, Indianapolis, IN 46202, USA
* Corresponding author.
E-mail address: jsfuqua@iu.edu

Endocrinol Metab Clin N Am 53 (2024) 251–265
https://doi.org/10.1016/j.ecl.2024.01.006
0889-8529/24/© 2024 Elsevier Inc. All rights reserved.
endo.theclinics.com

Table 1 Causes of peripheral precocious puberty	
Congenital PPP	CAH
	MAS
	Familial male-limited precocious puberty
	GR
Acquired PPP	Gonadal sex cord stromal tumors
	Granulosa cell tumor
	Sertoli-Leydig cell tumor
	Sex cord stromal tumor with annular tubules
	Thecal cell tumor
	Large cell calcifying Sertoli tumor
	Leydig cell tumor
	Mixed germ cell/sex cord tumors
	Gonadoblastoma
	ACT
	hCG-producing tumors
	Germ cell tumors
	Hepatoma
	Infantile choriocarcinoma
	VWGS
	Exogenous sex steroid exposure
	Ovarian cyst

Abbreviations: ACT, adrenocortical tumor; CAH, congenital adrenal hyperplasia; GR, glucocorticoid resistance; hCG, human chorionic gonadotropin; MAS, McCune-Albright syndrome; PPP, peripheral precocious puberty: VWGS, Van Wyk-Grumbach syndrome.

gonadotropins. However, because gonadotropin secretion is suppressed in PPP, these disorders feature little to no change in the prepuberal testis or the occurrence of testicular asymmetry. In girls, some cases of PPP may be difficult to distinguish from CPP. Some distinguishing features may include isolated virilization, vaginal bleeding with minimal breast development, or associated abnormalities such as café au lait macules, abdominal masses, or signs of hypothyroidism. The clinician should take care to distinguish benign variants, such as premature thelarche and premature adrenarche, from the more serious and progressive disorders of PPP. See Paul Kaplowitz and Peter A. Lee's article, "Females with Breast Development Before Three Years of Age," in this issue and Paul B Kaplowitz's article, "Premature pubarche: A pragmatic approach," in this issue for discussion of these conditions.

Congenital Causes of Peripheral Precocious Puberty

There are 4 etiologies of PPP that are caused by mutations in specific genes and result in abnormal sex steroid production during the prepubertal years (**Table 2**). All are rare, and a positive family history may or may not be present. The clinical manifestations of these conditions can be quite dramatic or relatively subtle. The pathophysiologic basis for all of them is complex and fascinating. Each of these disorders will be discussed individually in the following sections.

Congenital adrenal hyperplasia

Congenital adrenal hyperplasia (CAH) refers to a group of disorders that have in common an enzymatic block in the cortisol biosynthetic pathway. The most common form of CAH is 21-hydroxylase (21OHase) deficiency, which accounts for ~95% of cases. Therefore, for the purposes of this review, the terms CAH and 21OHase deficiency will

Table 2
Genetic causes of peripheral precocious puberty

Condition	Cause	Affected Gene	Mode of Inheritance	Presentation (Girls)	Presentation (Boys)	Treatment	Key Laboratory Finding	Other
Non-Classic CAH	Deficiency of 21-hydroxylase enzyme leading to a block in cortisol biosynthesis	CYP21A2	Autosomal recessive	Pubic and axillary hair, adult body odor, ± acne, and growth acceleration	Pubic and axillary hair, adult body odor, ± acne, and growth acceleration	Glucocorticoid, usually hydrocortisone	Elevated 17OHP and androgens	Bone age may be advanced
MAS	Activating mutation in the stimulatory subunit of the G-protein complex, Gsα	GNAS	Sporadic, Postzygotic	Sudden onset painless vaginal bleeding with minimal breast enlargement due to large unilateral ovarian cysts	Secondary sexual development with mildly enlarged testes, may have unilateral macro-orchidism	Girls: tamoxifen or letrozole Boys: bicalutamide plus anastrozole or letrozole	Elevated sex steroids, suppressed gonadotropins	Mosaic distribution of affected cells and within affected tissues
FMPP	Activating mutation in the LH receptor	LHCGR	Autosomal dominant (sex-limited) or sporadic	Unaffected	Secondary sexual development with mildly enlarged testes	Bicalutamide plus anastrozole or letrozole	Elevated testosterone, suppressed gonadotropins	Advanced bone age and linear growth acceleration
GR	Loss-of-function mutation in the glucocorticoid receptor	NR3C1	Familial or Sporadic	Pubic and axillary hair, adult body odor, and acne	Pubic and axillary hair, adult body odor, and acne	Dexamethasone	Elevated androgens, cortisol, and ACTH	Bone age may be advanced, no signs of Cushing syndrome

Abbreviations: 17OHP, 17-hydroxyprogesterone; ACTH, adrenocorticotropic hormone; CAH, congenital adrenal hyperplasia; FMPP, familial male-limited precocious puberty; GR, glucocorticoid resistance; LH, luteinizing hormone; MAS, McCune-Albright syndrome.

be used interchangeably. The underlying cause of CAH is a mutation in the *CYP21A2* gene, which encodes for the 21OHase enzyme. Because the condition is autosomal recessive, an individual needs to harbor a mutation on both copies of the *CYP21A2* gene in order to have the disease. Many different mutations of this gene have been identified, which lead to disparate degrees of deficiency of the 21OHase enzyme. This molecular heterogeneity in turn results in a broad spectrum of clinical signs and symptoms.[1]

The hypothalamic-pituitary-adrenal axis is exquisitely sensitive to a subnormal concentration of cortisol. In response to the lack of negative feedback, there is an outpouring of corticotrophin releasing hormone (CRH) and adrenocorticotropic hormone (ACTH). In the presence of the enzymatic block, the molecular precursors to cortisol accumulate and are diverted down the adrenal androgen pathway. Therefore, the clinical consequences of CAH result from excess androgen exposure. "Classic" CAH refers to severe forms of the disease and is typically diagnosed at birth through newborn screening, a salt-wasting crisis, or typical physical findings. The term "nonclassic" CAH (NCCAH, also termed "late-onset") is reserved for milder forms and is the only type of CAH that will be considered here. The prevalence of NCCAH varies widely by race and ethnicity and is most common in Whites and in people of Ashkenazi, Yugoslavian, Sicilian, and Yupik Indian extraction.[2]

Presentation. The cardinal features of NCCAH include early onset of pubic and axillary hair in addition to adult body odor ± acne in both boys and girls. Skeletal maturation as assessed by bone age radiographs is typically advanced, and linear growth acceleration may be present. Testicular volume is prepubertal in boys, and mild clitoromegaly may be present in girls.

Diagnosis. The diagnosis of CAH rests on an elevated serum 17-hydroxyprogesterone (17OHP) concentration. In equivocal cases, an ACTH stimulation test may confirm the diagnosis.[3] Genetic testing is optional but can be helpful in pinpointing the precise *CYP21A2* variant. In most cases, both parents are carriers for CAH, and there is a 25% chance of each offspring being affected.

Treatment. The decision of whether to treat a child with NCCAH requires careful consideration of risks and benefits.[4] Factors to consider include the degree of symptoms, absolute height, rate of bone age advancement, and predicted adult height. The major downside to treatment is iatrogenic adrenal insufficiency. Treatment consists of a glucocorticoid, usually hydrocortisone given 2 or 3 times a day. Parents and caregivers need to be educated on the importance of giving stress steroids during times of illness and injury. In many cases, treatment can be discontinued when children have reached their adult height.[5]

McCune-Albright syndrome

McCune-Albright syndrome (MAS) is a pleotropic disease that is often present in the form of a classic triad of precocious puberty, fibrous dysplasia of bone, and café au lait skin pigmentation. The condition is caused by a gain-of-function mutation in the *GNAS* gene, which encodes for the stimulatory subunit of the heterotrimeric G-protein complex known as Gs alpha (Gsα). In the presence of the mutation, the G-protein-mediated intracellular signaling pathway becomes constitutively activated, which in turn leads to downstream gene transcription. Because the receptors through which many hormones exert their effect are G-protein coupled, endocrine tissues are particularly at risk for involvement in MAS. The mutation that causes the disease arises in a postzygotic cell line and resides in a mosaic distribution within affected tissues.[6]

Therefore, both the severity of the condition and the specific manifestations vary widely between patients. The greatest source of morbidity in MAS is the bone disease, which can lead to fractures, bone pain, and deformity. However, here we will review only the aspects of the condition that relate to precocious puberty.

Presentation. The precocious puberty that occurs in MAS is far more common in girls than in boys and can arise as early as the first year of life. It typically presents as sudden onset of painless vaginal bleeding along with minimal breast development.[7] Additional findings include estrogenized vaginal mucosa, ± signs of adrenarche such as pubic hair, and ± café au lait pigmentation that has irregular borders and usually respects the midline. A large unilateral ovarian cyst and endometrial stripe are typically seen on pelvic ultrasound. In boys, the precocious puberty of MAS is typified by pubic and axillary hair, adult body odor, and enlargement of the penis. As in other forms of PPP in boys, the testicular volume is in a prepubertal or only slightly pubertal size range. Because the precocious puberty in MAS has an abrupt onset, the linear growth rate and bone age are often initially normal. Asymmetry of the face and/or other areas of the body may sometimes be appreciated.

Diagnosis. Due to the mosaic nature of the disease, the search for a *GNAS* mutation in peripheral blood is of low yield.[8] Therefore, the diagnosis of MAS is primarily clinical. Biochemical studies typically reveal extreme elevations in serum estradiol (girls) or testosterone (boys) along with suppressed gonadotropins. A meticulous physical examination may show café au lait pigmentation (**Fig. 1**), laboratory studies assess for endocrine hyperfunction (beyond precocious puberty), and a bone scan screens for fibrous dysplasia. Forme fruste cases of MAS are common in which only 1 or 2 of the classic trial, or atypical combinations of features, are present. Failure to recognize the possibility of MAS in young girls with vaginal bleeding and an ovarian "mass" may lead to unnecessary oophorectomy.[9]

Treatment. The precocious puberty of MAS is intermittent and unpredictable. Long intervals of quiescence can last for years between episodes of vaginal bleeding. Therefore, a period of watchful waiting is recommended prior to embarking on treatment. In the subset of girls who have frequent bouts of autonomous ovarian function and bleeding, options include the selective estrogen receptor modulator tamoxifen or the third-generation aromatase inhibitor (AI), letrozole. Limited prospective and retrospective studies have suggested that both are safe and satisfactorily effective but no large-scale controlled studies have been conducted with either.[10,11] State-of-the-art

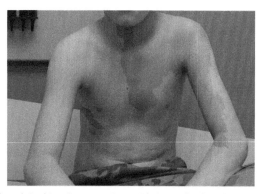

Fig. 1. Typical café au lait skin pigmentation with irregular borders in a child with MAS.

treatment of precocious puberty in boys uses an androgen receptor blocker, such as bicalutamide, and an AI such as anastrozole or letrozole.[12]

Familial male precocious puberty (also known as testotoxicosis)
Familial male precocious puberty (FMPP) is an uncommon form of PPP that occurs only in boys. It is caused by an activating mutation in the *LHCGR* gene, which encodes the LH receptor, resulting in autonomous testosterone production by the testicular Leydig cells. It is inherited in an autosomal dominant fashion but can also arise through a de novo mutation.[13] An important clue for FMPP is a family history of men with heights shorter than their genetic potential. Although mothers can transmit the disorder to their sons, FMPP is not expressed in women. This is because both follicle stimulating hormone (FSH) *and* luteinizing hormone (LH) are required for ovarian estrogen production.

Presentation. Boys with FMPP usually come to medical attention between ages 2 and 6 years. They present with phallic enlargement, pubic and axillary hair, adult body odor, acne, and linear growth acceleration. Their testicular volumes are disproportionately small ($< \sim 6$ cc) compared with the degree of virilization. Bone age is significantly advanced. In addition to their physical changes, parents may report increased aggression and inappropriate sexual acting out.

Diagnosis. Testing includes measurement of androgens and gonadotropins, along with a bone age radiograph. Testosterone concentrations in boys with FMPP are typically greater than 100 ng/dL, and gonadotropins are suppressed. The diagnosis may be confirmed through genetic testing of the *LHCGR* gene. The most common mutation is the substitution of aspartate for glycine at position 578.[14]

Treatment. The mainstay of treatment in boys with FMPP consists of an androgen receptor blocker and an AI.[15] Current treatment consists of bicalutamide with anastrozole or letrozole.[16] Long-term treatment results in an adult height that is normal for the general population although slightly less than the midparental height. A gonadotropin releasing hormone agonist (GnRHa) may be added if secondary CPP occurs. Intriguingly, spontaneous remission with normal adult height has been reported in a male family member harboring the same mutation as an affected proband.[17] A waxing and waning course in a child with genetically confirmed FMPP has also been reported.[18] This suggests the presence of modifier genes or other factors that can alter the phenotypic expression of the mutation.

Glucocorticoid resistance
Glucocorticoid resistance (GR), also known as Chrousos syndrome, is a rare disorder caused by an inactivating mutation in the glucocorticoid receptor, rendering it resistant to cortisol. The result is an inability of glucocorticoids to exert their normal effects at the level of the tissues. There is a compensatory increase in circulating cortisol and ACTH with a subsequent elevation of adrenal androgens and mineralocorticoids. The condition is heterogeneous and may be familial or sporadic. Complete unresponsiveness to glucocorticoids is thought to be incompatible with life. Therefore, all cases of GR are partial. Only those aspects of the condition that relate to PPP will be considered here.

Presentation. GR-induced PPP leads to symptoms of androgen exposure. Thus, boys and girls present with early onset of pubic and axillary hair, adult body odor, and acne.[19] Linear growth acceleration and bone age advancement may also occur. Testicular volume in boys will be small. Despite the high serum concentrations of cortisol, features of Cushing syndrome are absent. GR has been identified as a cause for premature pubarche in a child aged as young as 2 years[20] and implicated as the cause for precocious puberty with galactorrhea in a 7-year-old child.[21]

Diagnosis. In patients with suspected GR, a careful history including family history and physical examination looking for evidence of mineralocorticoid and/or androgen excess is the first step. Biochemical testing should include serum androgens as well as cortisol and ACTH. A 24-hour urinary free cortisol on 2 or 3 successive days is also recommended.[22] Definitive diagnosis rests on molecular genetic analysis of *NR3C1*, the gene encoding the glucocorticoid receptor. Thus far, 31 different gene mutations in this receptor have been identified.[23] The greatest diagnostic challenge in GR is a failure to consider this uncommon entity in children presenting with hyperandrogenism.

Treatment. The goal of treatment in GR is to lower ACTH concentrations to halt excess production of androgens. This is accomplished with mineralocorticoid-sparing glucocorticoids such as dexamethasone. In children, this results in the prevention of further secondary sexual development and a gradual improvement in the ratio of bone age to chronologic age.

Acquired Causes of Peripheral Precocious Puberty

In addition to syndromic PPP with genetic causes, there are a host of acquired conditions that may lead to PPP. These include tumors of the gonads, adrenal glands, or other tissues; PPP associated with severe hypothyroidism; exogenous sex steroid exposure; and ovarian cysts.

Tumors causing peripheral precocious puberty

Certain tumors may produce sex hormones directly, whereas others may release human chorionic gonadotropin (hCG) that causes sex hormone secretion from normal gonads. Because some tumors are masculinizing and others feminizing, the associated physical changes may not necessarily align with the patient's sex. We will first describe the pathophysiology and clinical presentation of gonadal tumors and then review adrenal tumors and other tumors of non-steroid-producing tissues.

Gonadal tumors

Sex Cord Stromal Tumors Sex cord stromal tumors are rare neoplasms that arise from the nongerm cell components of the gonads. They can occur in both male and female individuals. Sex cord stromal tumors differ from germ cell-derived tumors in that they are often secretory, producing testosterone or estradiol depending on the tumor subtype.

Juvenile granulosa cell tumors (JGCTs) secrete estrogen and are the most common pediatric sex cord stromal tumor. There is little distinction between granulosa cell tumors and granulosa-thecal cell tumors. JGCTs typically present in adolescence and young adulthood but may occur as early as 6 months of age and present with precocious puberty.[24] In postmenarchal girls, JGCT may lead to menstrual irregularity, abdominal pain/distention, and an abdominal mass. On ultrasound, they appear as unilateral cystic or partially cystic masses ranging from 3 to 23 cm with a median size of 11 cm.[25] The tumors may secrete inhibin, which can be used as a tumor marker. Treatment is primarily surgical, although chemotherapy may be required. The prognosis is excellent.

Sertoli-Leydig cell tumors arise in the ovary. They typically occur in the first 3 decades of life. Histologically, they include tubular structures containing Sertoli cells with intervening areas containing clusters of Leydig cells. The tumors are often nonsecretory but may produce androgens or sometimes estrogens. Presenting findings typically include abdominal pain, distention, and a palpable mass but signs of virilization, breast development, and vaginal bleeding may also occur.[26] Poorly differentiated Sertoli-Leydig cell tumors are often associated with *DICER1* mutations. The DICER1 protein is critical for gene transcription, and Sertoli-Leydig cell tumors may occur in association with pleuropulmonary blastoma, thyroid nodules or carcinoma, cystic nephroma, and other tumors.[27] Treatment of Sertoli-Leydig cell tumors is primarily surgical. Adjuvant chemotherapy is usually recommended for higher stage tumors.[28]

Sex cord stromal tumors with annular tubules occur in ovaries and may be associated with Peutz-Jeghers syndrome. They are usually unilateral but may be bilateral. Histologically, they are characterized by round nests of cells surrounded by a hyalinized basement membrane, and they may secrete both estradiol and testosterone.[29] Patients usually present in adolescence or young adulthood with menstrual irregularity but precocious puberty may also occur.[28] Peutz-Jeghers syndrome is caused by mutations in the *STK11* gene and manifests as autosomally dominantly inherited mucocutaneous pigmentation and gastrointestinal hamartomas. Malignancies of the gastrointestinal tract, breast, ovaries, cervix, and testes also occur as part of this syndrome.

Thecal cell tumors (thecomas) are very rare, usually benign, and occur primarily in older women. A subset of thecomas, called luteinized thecomas, occurs in younger women and occasionally in children and adolescents. Luteinized thecomas produce estrogen in 50% of cases and androgen in 11%[30] and thus may lead to feminization or virilization.

Large-cell calcifying Sertoli cell tumors are rare testicular tumors that may occur in boys with Peutz-Jeghers syndrome as well as Carney complex and neurofibromatosis type 1. They most commonly present as an isolated testicular mass but may produce aromatase and secrete estradiol, leading to feminization with prepubertal gynecomastia and growth acceleration. Bilateral involvement occurs in 20% of cases and may make clinical detection difficult.[31] The majority of large-cell calcifying Sertoli cell tumors are benign.

Leydig cell tumors occur in the testes and cause virilization through secretion of testosterone. Boys with Leydig cell tumors present at a mean age of 6.5 years with signs of virilization, such as rapid linear growth, pubic hair, and penile enlargement.[32] Tumors are almost always unilateral and cause testicular asymmetry. Serum testosterone concentrations can range from undetectable to greater than 800 ng/dL.[32] Gonadotropins are typically suppressed but this may be incomplete based on the degree of aromatization of testosterone to estradiol.[32] Ultrasonography usually reveals a mass with hypoechoic to nearly isoechoic echotexture and variable margins with increased vascularity.[32,33] Treatment is usually testis-sparing surgery because Leydig cell tumors in children are universally benign.[34]

Mixed Germ Cell/Sex Cord Tumors *Gonadoblastomas* are benign tumors that typically arise in the setting of gonadal dysgenesis with a Y chromosome-bearing cell line. They are composed of a mixture of primitive germ cells and immature Sertoli or granulosa cells with occasional calcification.[35] Bilateral involvement is common. Presenting features may include abdominal pain or a palpable mass but gonadoblastomas may also secrete testosterone and cause virilization. Although gonadoblastomas most commonly present in adolescence and young adulthood, they may occur in younger children or even infants, especially in those with 46,XY gonadal dysgenesis. Although affected patients usually have genital ambiguity, some may be phenotypically female, such as those with complete gonadal dysgenesis (Swyer syndrome) or Turner syndrome with a Y chromosome cell line. Although pure gonadoblastomas are benign, in about 50% of cases, they occur in association with gonadal malignancies, especially dysgerminoma.[36] Dysgerminomas are usually nonsecretory but may rarely produce estradiol. Treatment is surgical resection.

Adrenocortical tumors. Adrenocortical tumors (ACTs) account for only 0.2% of childhood malignancies, with a worldwide annual incidence of 0.3 to 0.38 cases/million children aged younger than 15 years.[37,38] The average age of presentation in childhood is 3.8 years.[39] Ninety percent of ACTs in children are functional, usually producing androgens and/or glucocorticoids. Most patients present with either isolated virilization or a combination of virilization and Cushing syndrome. Findings may include rapid penile or clitoral enlargement, with acne, pubic hair, and rapid height gain. Boys will have prepubertal testes. Cushingoid changes may include rapid weight gain, striae, and moon facies.

The laboratory evaluation for virilizing ACTs typically reveals elevated serum testosterone, androstenedione, dehydroepiandrosterone sulfate (DHEA-S), high midnight salivary cortisol levels, lack of suppression of serum cortisol following dexamethasone, or elevated 24-hour urinary cortisol excretion. Imaging studies are required to localize the tumor and determine the extent of disease. Either MRI or computed tomography (CT) is acceptable for abdominal imaging, although CT is preferred for chest imaging.

It may be difficult to distinguish a benign adenoma from a malignant adrenocortical carcinoma, and there are various grading systems used for this purpose.[39]

Treatment of ACTs is surgical removal. All ACTs should be considered malignant at the time of surgery. Because of the friability and invasive nature of malignant tumors, the procedure is best done by experienced surgeons because tumor spillage during resection leads to a worse prognosis. Stage 1 tumors have a very good long-term prognosis, with more than 90% survival, although higher stage tumors have a progressively worse prognosis.[40] There is an increased incidence of ACTs in several inherited malignancy syndromes, including Li-Fraumeni syndrome, familial adenomatous polyposis, and Beckwith-Wiedemann syndrome.

Human chorionic gonadotropin-secreting tumors

Germ cell tumors Germ cell tumors account for 3% of all childhood malignancies.[41] Germ cell tumors can be divided into 2 groups: "pure" germinomas, which comprise 50% to 70% of the total and tend to occur in older children and adolescents, and nongerminomatous germ cell tumors (NGGCT), which comprise 30% and occur more often in younger children. The NGGCT category includes several histologic subtypes, such as teratomas, embryonal carcinomas, choriocarcinomas, yolk sac tumors, and tumors with mixed histologies. Germ cell tumors tend to produce high levels of hCG and alpha-fetoprotein.

Germ cell tumors lead to precocious puberty through the action of hCG, which binds to the LH receptor in testes and leads to GnRH-independent testosterone secretion. It thus affects male individuals almost exclusively.[42] Affected boys present with acne, pubic hair, penile growth, deepening of the voice, and increased height velocity. Testicular size is only slightly increased above prepubertal norms due to the lack of Sertoli cell and seminiferous tubule development. Gynecomastia may be present due to aromatization of high concentrations of testosterone.

Laboratory evaluation shows suppression of LH and FSH concentrations and elevated levels of hCG and alpha-fetoprotein. CNS imaging reveals germ cell tumors, most commonly located in the pineal or suprasellar regions. In addition to PPP, intracranial germ cell tumors may cause CPP in both boys and girls through their mass effect.[42] Extracranial germ cell tumors occur in the mediastinum, liver, or gonads. Twenty percent of patients with mediastinal germ cell tumors have Klinefelter syndrome.[43]

Germinomas are typically radiosensitive and carry a good prognosis. NGGCT typically require chemotherapy and have a worse prognosis.

Hepatoblastoma Hepatoblastoma is the most common primary liver cancer in children and occurs at a mean age of 18 months.[44] It is estimated that 100 new cases are diagnosed in the United States each year.[45] Hepatoblastomas are associated with several syndromes, including Beckwith-Wiedemann syndrome, familial adenomatous polyposis, and trisomy 18. The tumors secrete high levels of alpha-fetoprotein, and 18% also produce hCG.[46] Despite this, precocious puberty is only rarely seen, with about 40 cases reported in the literature.[46]

Patients with hepatoblastoma-associated precocious puberty are male infants, toddlers, and preschoolers. Presenting findings include hepatomegaly, palpable abdominal mass, penile enlargement, and pubic hair. Testicular volume is mildly increased. Laboratory studies show suppressed LH and FSH with high testosterone, hCG, and alpha-fetoprotein concentrations. Advances in preoperative neoadjuvant chemotherapy have increased survival rates to 70% to 80%.[47]

Infantile choriocarcinoma Infantile choriocarcinoma occurs in newborns and very young infants and is thought to be a complication of maternal placental choriocarcinoma during pregnancy. Patients present with anemia, failure to thrive, and hepatomegaly, and affected boys may have precocious puberty due to high concentrations of hCG. Infantile choriocarcinoma usually occurs in the liver, lung, or brain. It is rapidly fatal, and death occurs an average of 3 weeks after diagnosis.[48] The condition is treatable with chemotherapy, which improves survival if recognized early.

Van Wyk-Grumbach syndrome

First described in 1960, Van Wyk-Grumbach syndrome (VWGS), features pubertal changes in association with severe primary hypothyroidism. Girls with VWGS present with breast development, vaginal bleeding, and/or large ovarian cysts without pubic or axillary hair. Boys have isolated testicular enlargement without pubic and axillary hair or genital enlargement. Linear growth failure and significantly delayed bone ages are typical. Some children present with an abdominal mass due to large ovarian cysts, pituitary masses from thyrotrope hypertrophy, or short stature with unrecognized pubertal changes. In one series of 30 patients, the median age at presentation was 9 years, with a height SDS of −2.83, weight SDS of −0.94, and a mean bone age delay of 2.9 years.[49] The frequency of VWGS is not known with certainty, although one study suggested that it was present in as many as 24% of prepubertal-age children with serum TSH concentrations greater than 100 mU/L.[50] Failure to recognize the hypothyroidism may lead to unnecessary surgical intervention for supposed ovarian or testicular malignancy or pituitary tumor. Treatment of hypothyroidism leads to rapid advancement of bone age, which typically outpaces the increased height velocity and causes a permanent height deficit.

The cause of VWGS is not known with certainty. The clinical features suggest an FSH-mediated process, with stimulation of ovarian follicles and seminiferous tubule growth without thecal cell or Leydig cell stimulation. Indeed, FSH concentrations tend to be high, with normal prepubertal LH levels. Proposed mechanisms include an "overlap" stimulation of FSH secretion by elevated thyrotropin releasing hormone (TRH) concentrations or a cross-reactivity of TSH at the FSH receptor.[51]

Exogenous sex steroids

Many reports of exogenous estrogen-induced breast development in boys and girls have been published in the last 70 years, including oral and transdermal exposures. More recently, there have been reports of breast development from exposure to estrogen-containing hair care products and lavender and tea tree oils, which contain estrogenic and antiandrogenic compounds.[52,53]

Most recent reports of exogenous sex steroid-induced PPP have involved unintentional passage of transdermal testosterone from parent to child.[54] Findings may include pubic and axillary hair, penile or clitoral enlargement, acne, and accelerated growth. Laboratory testing may show elevated serum testosterone concentrations and gonadotropins may be suppressed or in the normal prepubertal range. Eliminating the exposure halts the progression of pubertal changes, although it may take weeks to months for the serum testosterone level to return to the normal range for age.[55,56]

In premarketing industry studies of a transdermal testosterone gel in which men applied the gel to their abdomens, 15 minutes of daily skin-to-skin contact with their female partners as much as quadrupled the women's testosterone levels.[57] Package inserts recommend handwashing and covering the exposed area with clothing.

Ovarian cysts

Autonomously functioning ovarian cysts are the most common estrogen-producing ovarian disease in children. Symptoms include rapidly progressive breast development, and menstrual bleeding often occurs early in the course. Estradiol levels may be low if the cyst has resolved but may be as high as 250 pg/mL. Baseline serum gonadotropin concentrations are suppressed or in the prepubertal range and do not respond to GnRH stimulation. Levels of testosterone and DHEA-S are usually normal, and bone age may be normal or advanced. Pelvic ultrasonography shows a unilateral ovarian cyst greater than 1 cm in diameter, and cysts can be 7 cm or more. Ovarian cysts are transient, and tumor markers such as hCG and inhibin B are normal.

The median time to resolution of autonomously functioning ovarian cysts in a study of 12 girls was 6 months, with a range of 2 to 13 months.[58] Other reports indicate shorter durations from 1 to 3 months.[59,60] Longer duration of cysts is associated with a higher risk of recurrence.[58]

SUMMARY

In conclusion, the extensive differential diagnosis of PPP includes congenital and acquired causes. Presenting features depend on which class of sex steroids is involved, and diagnosis rests on hormonal and, if indicated, imaging and/or genetic studies. Effective treatment exists for nearly all causes of PPP. Ongoing research will advance our therapeutic armamentarium and understanding of the pathophysiologic basis for PPP.

CLINICS CARE POINTS

- PPP can be due to exogenous exposure, tumor steroid production, or unregulated gonadal secretion.
- Hallmarks of MAS include café au lait pigmentation, fibrous dysplasia of bone, or intermittent breast development and early vaginal bleeding in girls.
- Boys with familial male-limited precocious puberty usually have a maternal family history of male early puberty or short stature.

- Boys with PPP have either prepubertal-sized testes, testes that are smaller than expected for the stage of puberty, or testicular asymmetry.
- Girls with ovarian tumors may present with palpable abdominal masses, breast development, and/or vaginal bleeding.
- Children with PPP due to VWGS may have pituitary hyperplasia that can be mistaken for a pituitary adenoma.

DISCLOSURE

The authors have nothing to disclose.

REFERENCES

1. Merke DP, Auchus RJ. Congenital adrenal hyperplasia due to 21-hydroxylase deficiency. N Engl J Med 2020;383(13):1248–61.
2. Hannah-Shmouni F, Morissette R, Sinaii N, et al. Revisiting the prevalence of non-classic congenital adrenal hyperplasia in US Ashkenazi Jews and Caucasians. Genet Med 2017;19(11):1276–9.
3. Turcu AF, El-Maouche D, Zhao L, et al. Androgen excess and diagnostic steroid biomarkers for nonclassic 21-hydroxylase deficiency without cosyntropin stimulation. Eur J Endocrinol 2020;183(1):63–71.
4. Claahsen-van der Grinten HL, Speiser PW, Ahmed SF, et al. Congenital adrenal hyperplasia-current insights in pathophysiology, diagnostics, and management. Endocr Rev 2022;43(1):91–159.
5. Nebesio TD, Eugster EA. Growth and reproductive outcomes in congenital adrenal hyperplasia. Int J Pediatr Endocrinol 2010;2010:298937.
6. Boyce AM, Collins MT. Fibrous dysplasia/mccune-albright syndrome: a rare, mosaic disease of galpha s activation. Endocr Rev 2020;41(2):345–70.
7. Tufano M, Ciofi D, Amendolea A, et al. Auxological and endocrinological features in children with mccune albright syndrome: a review. Front Endocrinol 2020;11:522.
8. Gryngarten M, Comar H, Arcari A, et al. McCune-Albright syndrome, a rare form of precocious puberty: Diagnosis, treatment, and follow-up. Arch Argent Pediatr 2021;119(5):e420–7.
9. Nabhan ZM, West KW, Eugster EA. Oophorectomy in McCune-Albright syndrome: a case of mistaken identity. J Pediatr Surg 2007;42(9):1578–83.
10. de GBPC, Kuperman H, Cabral de Menezes-Filho H, et al. Tamoxifen improves final height prediction in girls with mccune-albright syndrome: a long follow-up. Horm Res Paediatr 2015;84(3):184–9.
11. Estrada A, Boyce AM, Brillante BA, et al. Long-term outcomes of letrozole treatment for precocious puberty in girls with McCune-Albright syndrome. Eur J Endocrinol 2016;175(5):477–83.
12. Neyman A, Eugster EA. Treatment of girls and boys with mccune-albright syndrome with precocious puberty - update 2017. Pediatr Endocrinol Rev 2017; 15(2):136–41.
13. Themmen AP, Martens JW, Brunner HG. Activating and inactivating mutations in LH receptors. Mol Cell Endocrinol 1998;145(1–2):137–42.
14. Kremer H, Martens JW, van Reen M, et al. A limited repertoire of mutations of the luteinizing hormone (LH) receptor gene in familial and sporadic patients with male LH-independent precocious puberty. J Clin Endocrinol Metab 1999;84(3): 1136–40.

15. Schoelwer M, Eugster EA. Treatment of Peripheral Precocious Puberty. Endocr Dev 2016;29:230–9.
16. Reiter EO, Mauras N, McCormick K, et al. Bicalutamide plus anastrozole for the treatment of gonadotropin-independent precocious puberty in boys with testotoxicosis: a phase II, open-label pilot study (BATT). J Pediatr Endocrinol Metab 2010;23(10):999–1009.
17. Kreher NC, Pescovitz OH, Delameter P, et al. Treatment of familial male-limited precocious puberty with bicalutamide and anastrozole. J Pediatr 2006;149(3):416–20.
18. Nabhan ZM, Eugster EA. Testotoxicosis with an episodic course: an unusual case within a series. AACE Clin Case Rep 2019;5(1):e50–3.
19. Witchel SF, Smith RR. Glucocorticoid resistance in premature pubarche and adolescent hyperandrogenism. Mol Genet Metab 1999;66(2):137–41.
20. Nader N, Bachrach BE, Hurt DE, et al. A novel point mutation in helix 10 of the human glucocorticoid receptor causes generalized glucocorticoid resistance by disrupting the structure of the ligand-binding domain. J Clin Endocrinol Metab 2010;95(5):2281–5.
21. Xiang SL, He LP, Ran XW, et al. [Primary glucocorticoid resistance syndrome presenting as pseudo-precocious puberty and galactorrhea]. Sichuan Da Xue Xue Bao Yi Xue Ban 2008;39(5):861–4.
22. Nicolaides NC, Kino T, Chrousos G, et al. Primary generalized glucocorticoid resistance or chrousos syndrome. In: Feingold KR, Anawalt B, Blackman MR, et al, editors. Endotext. South Dartmouth, MA: MDText.com, Inc.; 2000.
23. Huang H, Wang W. Molecular mechanisms of glucocorticoid resistance. Eur J Clin Invest 2023;53(2):e13901.
24. Hansen R, Lewis A, Sullivan C, et al. Juvenile granulosa cell tumor diagnosed in 6-month-old infant with precocious puberty. Radiol Case Rep 2021;16(9):2609–13.
25. Fresneau B, Orbach D, Faure-Conter C, et al. Sex-cord stromal tumors in children and teenagers: results of the TGM-95 study. Pediatr Blood Cancer 2015;62(12):2114–9.
26. Hendricks M, Cois A, Geel J, et al. Sex cord stromal tumors in children and adolescents: a first report by the south african children's cancer study group (1990-2015). J Pediatr Hematol Oncol 2021;43(5):e619–24.
27. Gonzalez IA, Stewart DR, Schultz KAP, et al. DICER1 tumor predisposition syndrome: an evolving story initiated with the pleuropulmonary blastoma. Mod Pathol 2022;35(1):4–22.
28. Schneider DT, Orbach D, Ben-Ami T, et al. Consensus recommendations from the EXPeRT/PARTNER groups for the diagnosis and therapy of sex cord stromal tumors in children and adolescents. Pediatr Blood Cancer 2021;68(Suppl 4):e29017.
29. Bhardwaj S, Kalir T. Gynecologic manifestations of Peutz-Jeghers syndrome. Int J Gynecol Cancer 2023;33(4):640–2.
30. Zhang J, Young RH, Arseneau J, et al. Ovarian stromal tumors containing lutein or Leydig cells (luteinized thecomas and stromal Leydig cell tumors)–a clinicopathological analysis of fifty cases. Int J Gynecol Pathol 1982;1(3):270–85.
31. Gourgari E, Saloustros E, Stratakis CA. Large-cell calcifying Sertoli cell tumors of the testes in pediatrics. Curr Opin Pediatr 2012;24(4):518–22.
32. Olivier P, Simoneau-Roy J, Francoeur D, et al. Leydig cell tumors in children: contrasting clinical, hormonal, anatomical, and molecular characteristics in boys and girls. J Pediatr 2012;161(6):1147–52.

33. Tsitouridis I, Maskalidis C, Panagiotidou D, et al. Eleven patients with testicular leydig cell tumors: clinical, imaging, and pathologic correlation. J Ultrasound Med 2014;33(10):1855–64.

34. Miao X, Li Y, Zhou T, et al. Testis-sparing surgery in children with testicular tumors: A systematic review and meta-analysis. Asian J Surg 2021;44(12):1503–9.

35. Maleki Z, Loveless M, Fraig M. Coexistence of gonadoblastoma and dysgerminoma in a dysgenetic gonad on touch preparation: a case report. Diagn Cytopathol 2011;39(1):42–4.

36. Chandrapattan P, Jena A, Patnayak R, et al. Gonadoblastoma with dysgerminoma presenting as virilizing disorder in a young child with 46, XX karyotype: a case report and review of the literature. Case Rep Endocrinol 2022;2022: 5666957.

37. Brondani VB, Fragoso M. Pediatric adrenocortical tumor - review and management update. Curr Opin Endocrinol Diabetes Obes 2020;27(3):177–86.

38. Faria AM, Almeida MQ. Differences in the molecular mechanisms of adrenocortical tumorigenesis between children and adults. Mol Cell Endocrinol 2012; 351(1):52–7.

39. Fuqua JS. Adrenal Tumors in Childhood. Adv Pediatr 2021;68:227–44.

40. Ribeiro RC, Pinto EM, Zambetti GP, et al. The International Pediatric Adrenocortical Tumor Registry initiative: contributions to clinical, biological, and treatment advances in pediatric adrenocortical tumors. Mol Cell Endocrinol 2012;351(1): 37–43.

41. Kaatsch P, Hafner C, Calaminus G, et al. Pediatric germ cell tumors from 1987 to 2011: incidence rates, time trends, and survival. Pediatrics 2015;135(1):e136–43.

42. Chen H, Ni M, Xu Y, et al. Precocious puberty due to intracranial germ cell tumors: a case-control study. Endocr Relat Cancer 2022;29(10):581–8.

43. Nichols CR. Mediastinal germ cell tumors. clinical features and biologic correlates. Chest 1991;99(2):472–9.

44. Eren E, Demirkaya M, Cakir ED, et al. A rare cause of precocious puberty: hepatoblastoma. J Clin Res Pediatr Endocrinol 2009;1(6):281–3.

45. Spector LG, Birch J. The epidemiology of hepatoblastoma. Pediatr Blood Cancer 2012;59(5):776–9.

46. Yhoshu E, Lone YA, Mahajan JK, et al. Hepatoblastoma with precocious puberty. J Indian Assoc Pediatr Surg 2019;24(1):68–71.

47. Sharma D, Subbarao G, Saxena R. Hepatoblastoma. Semin Diagn Pathol 2017; 34(2):192–200.

48. Blohm ME, Gobel U. Unexplained anaemia and failure to thrive as initial symptoms of infantile choriocarcinoma: a review. Eur J Pediatr 2004;163(1):1–6.

49. Kusuma Boddu S, Ayyavoo A, Hebbal Nagarajappa V, et al. Van wyk grumbach syndrome and ovarian hyperstimulation in juvenile primary hypothyroidism: lessons from a 30-case cohort. J Endocr Soc 2023;7(6):bvad042.

50. Cabrera SM, DiMeglio LA, Eugster EA. Incidence and characteristics of pseudoprecocious puberty because of severe primary hypothyroidism. J Pediatr 2013; 162(3):637–9.

51. Anasti JN, Flack MR, Froehlich J, et al. A potential novel mechanism for precocious puberty in juvenile hypothyroidism. J Clin Endocrinol Metab 1995;80(1): 276–9.

52. Ramsey JT, Li Y, Arao Y, et al. Lavender products associated with premature thelarche and prepubertal gynecomastia: case reports and endocrine-disrupting chemical activities. J Clin Endocrinol Metab 2019;104(11):5393–405.

53. Zimmerman PA, Francis GL, Poth M. Hormone-containing cosmetics may cause signs of early sexual development. Mil Med 1995;160(12):628–30.
54. Ramos CO, Macedo DB, Bachega T, et al. Premature pubarche due to exogenous testosterone gel or intense diaper rash prevention cream use: a case series. Horm Res Paediatr 2019;91(6):411–5.
55. Kunz GJ, Klein KO, Clemons RD, et al. Virilization of young children after topical androgen use by their parents. Pediatrics 2004;114(1):282–4.
56. Sanderson E, Abraham MB, Joseph J, et al. Variable persistence of serum testosterone in infants and children exposed to topical testosterone. J Paediatr Child Health 2020;56(9):1464–7.
57. de Ronde W. Hyperandrogenism after transfer of topical testosterone gel: case report and review of published and unpublished studies. Hum Reprod 2009; 24(2):425–8.
58. Heo S, Shim YS, Lee HS, et al. Clinical course of peripheral precocious puberty in girls due to autonomous ovarian cysts. Clin Endocrinol 2023;100(1):29–35.
59. de Sousa G, Wunsch R, Andler W. Precocious pseudopuberty due to autonomous ovarian cysts: a report of ten cases and long-term follow-up. Hormones (Basel) 2008;7(2):170–4.
60. Rodriguez-Macias KA, Thibaud E, Houang M, et al. Follow up of precocious pseudopuberty associated with isolated ovarian follicular cysts. Arch Dis Child 1999;81(1):53–6.

Delayed Puberty Including Constitutional Delay

Differential and Outcome

Jennifer Harrington, MBBS, PhD[a,b,*]

KEYWORDS

- Delayed puberty • Hypogonadism • Constitutional delay of growth and puberty

KEY POINTS

- The traditional definition of delayed puberty is either the absence of testicular development in boys by 14 years or the absence of breast development in girls by 13 years, with ongoing debate about lowering these age thresholds.
- Constitutional delay of growth and puberty (CDGP) is the most common cause of delayed puberty in both sexes.
- There is an increased understanding of the heterogeneity in both clinical presentation and the genetics underpinning CDGP.
- Even with advances in genetics and new biochemical approaches, differentiating youth with CDGP from other causes of delayed puberty remains challenging.
- As an alternative to low-dose steroids, ongoing research looking at aromatase inhibitors may in time be an alternative management approach for youth with CDGP in whom medical intervention is wanted.

DEFINING DELAYED PUBERTY

Delayed puberty is one of the most common presentations seen by pediatric endocrinologists.[1] It is defined as the absence of clinical signs of activation of the hypothalamic-pituitary-gonadal (HPG) axis by an age that is greater than 2 to 2.5 standard deviations from the mean of the general population.[2,3] Using this criterion, the traditional definition for delayed puberty is the lack of testicular development of 4 mL or greater in boys by 14 years of age and absence of breast development by 13 years in girls. The development of pubic hair is not included in this definition because this usually represents adrenarche, which is independent of HPG axis activation. There have been calls to reduce the age threshold for defining delayed puberty (down to 12 years in girls and 13.5 years in boys), given secular trends of earlier

Funding/Support: No specific funding/support.
a Division of Endocrinology, Women's and Children's Health Network, Adelaide, Australia;
b Faculty of Health and Medical Sciences, University of Adelaide, Adelaide, Australia
* 72 King William Road, North Adelaide 5006, Australia.
E-mail address: jenny.harrington@sa.gov.au

Endocrinol Metab Clin N Am 53 (2024) 267–278
https://doi.org/10.1016/j.ecl.2024.01.007
0889-8529/24/Crown Copyright © 2024 Published by Elsevier Inc. All rights reserved.
endo.theclinics.com

pubertal onset in the general population.[4,5] This has not yet, however, reached consensus, with the majority of North American Pediatric Endocrinologists in a published survey, still utilizing the traditional definition.[6]

Although not captured by this traditional definition of delayed puberty, there are conditions that can present with normal age of pubertal onset but with subsequent stalling in ongoing development. Pubertal nomograms detailing rates of normal pubertal timing within the population have been proposed to help identify youth with stalled or slow pubertal development that may warrant further investigation.[7,8]

CAUSES OF DELAYED PUBERTY

Differentiating between the underlying causes for delayed puberty can be challenging, with significant overlap in clinical features and biochemistry investigations between the various causes. Constitutional delay of growth and puberty (CDGP), sometimes referred to as self-limited delayed puberty, is the most common cause of delayed puberty in both sexes.[8–10] It is however a diagnosis of exclusion, and the differential diagnoses need to be considered (**Fig. 1**). These can be grouped into 3 main categories.

- Functional hypogonadotropic hypogonadism (FHH) arising from a transient delay in maturation of the HPG axis with associated low gonadotropins secondary to chronic medical conditions or medication.
- Permanent hypogonadotropic hypogonadism (PHH) from both acquired and congenital causes.
- Hypergonadotropic hypogonadism characterized by elevated gonadotropin concentrations with low sex steroid levels due to primary gonadal insufficiency.

Constitutional Delay of Growth and Puberty

CDGP is a self-limited condition representing a physiologic delay in the activation of the HPG axis at the limits of the normal population spectrum. CDGP is also classically

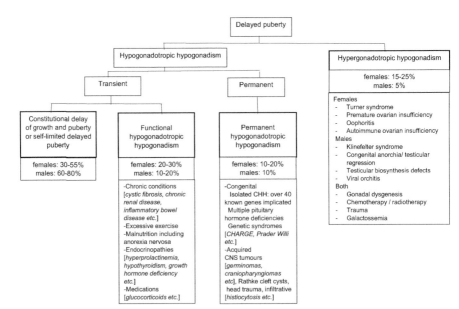

Fig. 1. Differential diagnostic categories for delayed puberty.

associated with slowing in growth that can affect final height.[11] It is increasingly appreciated, however, that youth with CDGP are a heterogeneous group; not all present with constitutional slowing in growth.[12] The term self-limited delayed puberty is therefore frequently being utilized instead of CDGP to encompass this heterogeneity, as well as youth in whom slow pubertal progression occurs, rather than delayed initiation. For simplicity, the term CDGP will be used in this article.

The timing of pubertal onset is a strongly inherited trait,[13] and similarly, CDGP has a strong genetic predisposition, with up to 50% to 75% of cases having a family history of delayed puberty.[14,15] CDGP also occurs more commonly in youth with a family history of congenital hypogonadotropic hypogonadism (CHH).[16] Genetic studies have not, however, empirically demonstrated common variants in genes associated with variations in pubertal timing in the majority of cases of CDGP.[17] Instead, an increasing number of distinct rare dominant gene defects have been described to occur in 7 to 25% of youth.[18–21]

Targeted and whole exome sequencing techniques have identified a variety of genetic variations to be associated with self-limited delayed puberty. These genes have a variety of different roles including modulating gonadotropin releasing hormone (GnRH) transcription (*EAP1*),[20] GnRH neural migration (*IGSF10*),[19] and development (*LGR4*).[22] There are also links between energy homeostasis and pubertal timing, with several genes involved in body mass regulation (*FTO* and *MC3R*)[21,23] found to be associated with CDGP. Although there is some overlap between genes involved with CHH (eg *HS6ST1*), other genes are quite distinct.[24]

Functional Hypogonadotropic Hypogonadism

Many different chronic conditions, as well as endocrinopathies, can result in an acquired, transient inhibition of the HPG axis, termed FHH (see **Fig. 1**). Common underlying pathways including malnutrition, hypercortisolemia, and proinflammatory cytokines are involved in the control of GnRH secretion,[25,26] leading to low gonadotropin concentrations. Intensive prolonged exercise, independent of body weight changes, also inhibits pulsatile GnRH secretion leading to pubertal arrest or delay.[27] There is, however, interindividual variability in the susceptibility of youth to develop delayed puberty to these stressors. Genetic susceptibility may have an important role in the manifestation of FHH, with higher rates of rare sequence variants in genes involved in HPG axis development and function found to be associated with hypothalamic amenorrhoea.[28]

Permanent Hypogonadotropic Hypogonadism

PHH arises from both acquired and congenital causes (see **Fig. 1**). There is increasing understanding of the genetic underpinnings of CHH, with causative genes found more than 50% of the time in cohorts.[17,29] For more detailed information on CHH and other forms of hypogonadotropic hypogonadism, the reader is referred to Krishna and colleagues' article, "Hypogonadotropic Hypogonadism," in this issue

Hypergonadotropic Hypogonadism

The final differential diagnostic category includes causes leading to primary gonadal failure or hypergonadotropic hypogonadism. In female individuals, Turner syndrome is the most common form of hypergonadotropic hypogonadism, with an incidence of 1 in 2000 to 2500 live female births.[30] Examples of other genetic causes include fragile X syndrome premutation carriers, galactosemia, and genes involved with gonadal dysgenesis. An increasing number of pathogenic genetic variants have been described in females with primary ovarian insufficiency, with whole exome or genome sequencing identifying the cause in approximately 30% of patients.[31]

In males, Klinefelter syndrome (47,XXY) is the most prevalent congenital cause of hypergonadotropic hypogonadism, although the majority of males present with stalled rather than delayed puberty. Additional examples of congenital causes include disorders of androgen biosynthesis, mutations in the luteinizing hormone (LH) and follicle stimulating hormone (FSH) receptor genes, and congenital anorchia. In both sexes, acquired cases of hypergonadotropic hypogonadism include among others, chemotherapy (particularly with alkylating agents), radiotherapy, trauma, and infections.

CLINICAL APPROACH TO THE DIAGNOSTIC WORKUP OF THE YOUTH WITH DELAYED PUBERTY

The goals in the diagnostic workup of the youth with delayed puberty are to identify in a timely manner the underlying cause, so that secondary underlying causes can be addressed and treatment initiated, particularly in those youth in whom there is an underlying organic cause. This can be challenging given the overlap in clinical presentation between the underlying diagnostic causes.

History and Examination

Key points in the history and examination that may help sway the diagnostic likelihood to one of the differential categories are outlined in **Table 1**. There is, however, still considerable overlap between diagnostic categories, especially when trying to differentiate between CDGP and CHH. Although more common in youth with CDGP, both may have a family history of delayed puberty.[32] Similarly, youth with CDGP compared to those with CHH have been demonstrated as a cohort to have lower mean height Z scores[32]; however, poor growth velocity is frequently a feature in patients with FHH as well. Compared with other diagnostic categories, the growth deceleration in children with CDGP tends to occur in the first 5 years of life.[33] Testicular volumes of 1 mL or less, as well as a history of bilateral cryptorchidism or micropenis, have strong specificity for CHH[9] but can also be features of hypergonadotropic hypogonadism such as in boys with Klinefelter syndrome. Further research evaluating integrated clinical scoring systems, along with biochemistry, is needed to aid in timely diagnosis.[32]

Investigations

Basal LH and FSH with the associated sex steroid (estrogen or early morning testosterone) concentrations are essential to identify patients with hypergonadotropic hypogonadism and should be tested in all youth with delayed puberty. Raised gonadotropins with low sex steroid levels are indicative of primary gonadal insufficiency. If found, subsequent testing then revolves around trying to identify the underlying cause, including karyotype plus any additional testing (such as fragile X testing) as indicated. Basal gonadotropins have not, however, been shown to be discriminatory between the other diagnostic categories,[34] as low LH concentrations occur both in transient and permanent forms of HPG axis inactivation.

Bone ages in children with delayed puberty are typically delayed, given the decreased sex hormone exposure to the epiphyses.[35] The degree of bone age delay between the diagnostic categories has not, however, been shown to be diagnostically discriminatory.[32] Bone age determination can still be useful in counseling about adult height prediction but has less value in the diagnostic workup.

In youth with low or prepubertal gonadotropins suggestive of either a transient or permanent form of hypogonadotropic hypogonadism, careful consideration of

Table 1
Discriminating features on history and physical examination between diagnostic categories

	CDGP	FHH	PHH	Hypergonadotropic Hypogonadism
History	Family history of delayed puberty History of decreased growth velocity (particularly between ages of 2 and 5 y)	Chronic disease Excessive exercise or weight-loss medications	Family history of delayed puberty History of CNS trauma, irradiation, etc. History suggestive of CNS pathology: headaches and visual changes Absent or decreased smell History of cryptorchidism History of renal agenesis, deafness, hand or feet anomalies, and skeletal anomalies	History of chemotherapy, gonadal radiotherapy, or trauma
Physical examination	Delayed adrenarche as well as pubarche	Low body mass index Growth velocity may be lower than normal prepubertal growth velocity range	Micropenis Testicular volume ≤1 mL Anosmia/hyposmia Bimanual synkinesia Adrenarche at normal age	Syndromic clinical features (eg, Turner or Klinefelter syndrome) Adrenarche at normal age

potential differentiating points on history and physical examination can help guide subsequent investigations (see **Table 1**, **Fig. 2**). Evidence of poor weight gain or abdominal symptoms should prompt consideration for screening for celiac or inflammatory bowel disease. A growth velocity less than 2 standard deviations for the bone age warrants testing insulin like growth factor 1 (IGF-1) levels as an initial workup for possible growth hormone deficiency. However, in the absence of any clinical features, wide screening biochemistry and hormone tests have low sensitivity in detecting an underlying organic cause of delayed puberty.[10]

MRI does have an important role, particularly as the chances of an organic cause become relatively larger the older the child is without signs of pubertal activation (see **Fig. 2**). MRI of the pituitary and olfactory bulbs can help to exclude an acquired form of hypogonadism (eg, central nervous system [CNS] tumor) or identify features of CHH (eg, absence of the olfactory bulbs and midline defects).

Differentiating between the causes of hypogonadotropic hypogonadism, particularly CHH and CDGP, in the absence of clinical clues, remains a challenge. Although CDGP can be diagnosed through clinical observation for evidence of spontaneous endogenous activation of the HPG axis before the age of 18 years, there have many efforts to identify discriminatory diagnostic tests to aid more timely diagnosis. Use of stimulation tests utilizing GnRH, GnRH agonists, or human chorionic gonadotropin has poor diagnostic discrimination.[34] Basal inhibin B concentrations are lower in youth with CHH compared to those in youth with CDGP[36] but there is significant overlap between diagnostic groups.[32,37] Subsequent approaches using GnRH agonist or FSH-stimulated inhibin B levels[38,39] as well as kisspeptin-stimulated LH concentrations have been proposed[40] but need further validation. To date therefore, there is not a reliable discriminatory biochemical diagnostic test to identify youth with CDGP.

As more genes are identified as leading to both CHH as well as CDGP, there are increasing calls to incorporate genetic panel testing into the routine diagnostic workup of the youth with delayed puberty.[41] When there are clinical features highly suggestive of CHH such as synkinesia or hypo/anosmia, genetic panels have relatively high rates of identifying underlying genetic causes.[42] In a cohort of 46 adolescents, only of 3 or whom had classic "red flags" for possible CHH, genetic panel testing

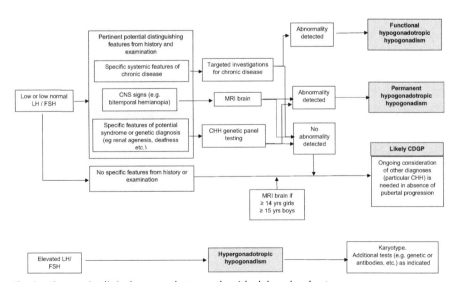

Fig. 2. Diagnostic clinical approach to youth with delayed puberty.

was able to identify a pathogenic variant in 33%,[41] supporting a more general use of this diagnostic test. Genetic panel testing does have its limitations. Selection of genes to be included on the panel is a balance between sensitivity and specificity; including a smaller number of highly causal genes or expanding inclusiveness to a larger number of possibly associated genes.[41] In addition, there remains a significant proportion of individuals with CHH in whom a genetic cause cannot be determined.[29,41] Genetic panel testing will continue to expand its diagnostic utility in the workup of the youth with delayed puberty but further research is still needed.

MANAGEMENT AND OUTCOME OF YOUTH WITH CONSTITUTIONAL DELAY OF GROWTH AND PUBERTY

In the youth with an underlying organic cause for pubertal delay, there are usually clear management pathways. When a diagnosis of FHH is made, the goal is to treat or address the underlying condition if possible. In PHH or hypergonadotropic hypogonadism, the traditional treatment involves sex steroid replacement, either in the form of testosterone or estrogen in titrating doses during a period of approximately 3 years until adult hormonal concentrations as well as full masculinization or feminization occur. There have been several reviews on this topic where this process is detailed.[3,43,44] In contrast, in youth in whom CDGP is suspected or if there is not yet a definitive diagnosis, navigating the management options versus expectant watching can be more challenging.

Given youth with CDGP should by definition have evidence of clinical pubertal onset by the age of 18 years, expectant observation may be sufficient management. Counseling families about when to expect spontaneous puberty onset to occur is difficult. A retrospective cohort of 97 girls and 243 boys with CDGP demonstrated a 62% chance for 13-year-old girls and 55% chance for 14-year-old boys to enter spontaneous puberty within the next year. This rate of pubertal progression is lower than would be expected using a normal distribution for pubertal onset.[45] The broad age range for pubertal entry means that a percentage of children may have to wait for quite a considerable time if interventions are not considered.

For a percentage of youth, CDGP is associated with an increased emotional distress. Studies have demonstrated mixed results, with some cohorts of youth with late pubertal onset having increased rates of depression and lower self-esteem,[46] with others not demonstrating differences in quality of life measures compared to controls.[47,48] Initiation of treatment to induce secondary sexual characteristics in male individuals has been shown to improve satisfaction with physical appearance using validated measures.[48]

The impact of associated short stature can, for a subset of adolescents with CDGP, be more distressing than the pubertal delay. Some studies have demonstrated that youth with CDGP have an attenuation in the growth potential, with an adult height on average of 4 cm lower when compared to midparental height.[11,49,50] Other studies have not demonstrated any impact on adult height,[51] likely reflecting the heterogeneous nature of CDGP.

Low-dose Sex Steroids

For those youth with delayed puberty where there is perceived distress or psychosocial challenges, many practitioners will offer a short-term course of low-dose sex steroids to induce secondary sexual characteristics and increase growth velocity. For male individuals, a typical management plan would involve monthly doses of 50 mg of an intramuscular testosterone ester for 3 months, with a further 3-month course up to 100 mg if there is no evidence of HPG activation (ie, testicular enlargement). At these doses, there are no adverse effects on adult height. A recent randomized study demonstrated that longer acting testosterone esters (testosterone undecanoate) at a dose of 250 mg every 3 months for 2 doses were comparable in terms of growth velocity and pubertal progression.[52] A proposed alternative is the use of daily testosterone gel (10 g daily).[53] In a retrospective study of 246 boys with delayed puberty comparing a 3-month course of intramuscular or transdermal testosterone to expectant observation, at 6 months, the boys receiving either testosterone treatment had a greater increase in growth velocity, with the transdermal group having the greatest increase compared to both other groups.[53] There have been reports of using oral testosterone for CDGP[8]; however, regional differences in availability of oral testosterone and the need to take multiple tablets twice a day may limit its usability.

For female individuals, there is a paucity of data on the use of low-dose estrogen in the management of CDGP. Typical protocols involve low-dose estrogen replacement with either 0.25 to 0.5 mg (or 5 μg/kg) of oral 17-β estradiol daily or 3.1 to 6.2 mcg/24 h (1/8–1/4 of 25 mcg/24 h patch) transdermal 17-β estradiol.[2,3,44] For both sexes, if there is no evidence of endogenous pubertal activation, the sex hormone doses will be gradually increased to full adult replacement. This would include the introduction of a progestin after 2 years of estrogen in any female individual with a uterus.

Alternate Management Options

Growth hormone is approved for the treatment of idiopathic short stature in certain countries, and these indications do not always implicitly exclude CDGP. There are minimal data supporting the effectiveness of growth hormone for CDGP.[3]

In male individuals with CDGP, there have been several small studies exploring the potential role of aromatase inhibitors such as letrozole. The potential advantages of letrozole would include delaying bone maturation through inhibiting the conversion of testosterone to estradiol and thus enhancing final adult height. It potentially could also help to induce activation of the HPG axis through decreasing the negative feedback loop from estradiol to the hypothalamus.[54] In a small randomized controlled study of 30 boys with CDGP comparing testosterone to letrozole, the letrozole group had greater testicular growth after 6 months.[55] There was, however, no difference in predicted adult height between groups. In contrast, a previous study demonstrated the combination of letrozole and testosterone resulted in a mean 5.1 cm improvement in predicted adult height.[56] Further data are needed on final adult height, as well as long-term safety data, before routine use of aromatase inhibitors in the management of boys with CDGP can be recommended.

SUMMARY

Of the past several years, there has been an increase in understanding of the underlying genetic interplay and heterogeneity in presentation of youth with CDGP. Although diagnosing CDGP in the absence of a clearly discriminatory test remains a challenge, future developments may help facilitate timely diagnoses, limit unnecessary tests, and guide appropriate management.

CLINICS CARE POINTS

- CDGP is the most common cause for delayed puberty in both male and female individuals but is a diagnosis of exclusion.

- CDGP is classically associated with a constitutional delay in growth in the first 5 years of life, delayed adrenarche, and a family history of delayed puberty.
- There currently is no one discriminatory test to distinguish CDGP from other causes of hypogonadotropic hypogonadism.
- There is increasing literature around the use of intramuscular and transdermal testosterone as well as aromatase inhibitors in male individuals with CDGP. There continues to be limited evidence for management options for female individuals.

DISCLOSURE

The author has no conflicts of interest to disclose.

REFERENCES

1. Bellotto E, Monasta L, Pellegrin MC, et al. Pattern and Features of Pediatric Endocrinology Referrals: A Retrospective Study in a Single Tertiary Center in Italy. Front Pediatr 2020;8:580588.
2. Harrington J, Palmert MR. An Approach to the Patient With Delayed Puberty. J Clin Endocrinol Metab 2022;107(6):1739–50.
3. Palmert MR, Dunkel L. Clinical practice. Delayed puberty. N Engl J Med 2012; 366(5):443–53.
4. Aksglaede L, Sorensen K, Petersen JH, et al. Recent decline in age at breast development: the Copenhagen Puberty Study. Pediatrics 2009;123(5):e932–9.
5. Sorensen K, Aksglaede L, Petersen JH, et al. Recent changes in pubertal timing in healthy Danish boys: associations with body mass index. J Clin Endocrinol Metab 2010;95(1):263–70.
6. Zhu J, Feldman HA, Eugster EA, et al. Practice Variation in the Management of Girls and Boys with Delayed Puberty. Endocr Pract 2020;26(3):267–84.
7. Lindhardt Johansen M, Hagen CP, Mieritz MG, et al. Pubertal Progression and Reproductive Hormones in Healthy Girls With Transient Thelarche. J Clin Endocrinol Metab 2017;102(3):1001–8.
8. Lawaetz JG, Hagen CP, Mieritz MG, et al. Evaluation of 451 Danish boys with delayed puberty: diagnostic use of a new puberty nomogram and effects of oral testosterone therapy. J Clin Endocrinol Metab 2015;100(4):1376–85.
9. Varimo T, Miettinen PJ, Kansakoski J, et al. Congenital hypogonadotropic hypogonadism, functional hypogonadotropism or constitutional delay of growth and puberty? An analysis of a large patient series from a single tertiary center. Hum Reprod 2017;32(1):147–53.
10. Abitbol L, Zborovski S, Palmert MR. Evaluation of delayed puberty: what diagnostic tests should be performed in the seemingly otherwise well adolescent? Arch Dis Child 2016;101(8):767–71.
11. Rohani F, Alai MR, Moradi S, et al. Evaluation of near final height in boys with constitutional delay in growth and puberty. Endocr Connect 2018;7(3):456–9.
12. Zhu J, Liu E, Feld A, et al. Approaches to Identify Factors Associated with Pubertal Timing in Self-Limited Delayed Puberty. Horm Res Paediatr 2023;96(3): 267–77.
13. Morris DH, Jones ME, Schoemaker MJ, et al. Familial concordance for age at menarche: analyses from the Breakthrough Generations Study. Paediatr Perinat Epidemiol 2011;25(3):306–11.

14. Zhu J, Choa RE, Guo MH, et al. A shared genetic basis for self-limited delayed puberty and idiopathic hypogonadotropic hypogonadism. J Clin Endocrinol Metab 2015;100(4):E646–54.
15. Busch AS, Hagen CP, Juul A. Heritability of pubertal timing: detailed evaluation of specific milestones in healthy boys and girls. Eur J Endocrinol 2020;183(1): 13–20.
16. Sedlmeyer IL, Hirschhorn JN, Palmert MR. Pedigree analysis of constitutional delay of growth and maturation: determination of familial aggregation and inheritance patterns. J Clin Endocrinol Metab 2002;87(12):5581–6.
17. Cassatella D, Howard SR, Acierno JS, et al. Congenital hypogonadotropic hypogonadism and constitutional delay of growth and puberty have distinct genetic architectures. Eur J Endocrinol 2018;178(4):377–88.
18. Barroso PS, Jorge AAL, Lerario AM, et al. Clinical and Genetic Characterization of a Constitutional Delay of Growth and Puberty Cohort. Neuroendocrinology 2020; 110(11–12):959–66.
19. Howard SR, Guasti L, Ruiz-Babot G, et al. IGSF10 mutations dysregulate gonadotropin-releasing hormone neuronal migration resulting in delayed puberty. EMBO Mol Med 2016;8(6):626–42.
20. Mancini A, Howard SR, Cabrera CP, et al. EAP1 regulation of GnRH promoter activity is important for human pubertal timing. Hum Mol Genet 2019;28(8):1357–68.
21. Duckett K, Williamson A, Kincaid JWR, et al. Prevalence of deleterious variants in MC3R in patients with constitutional delay of growth and puberty. J Clin Endocrinol Metab 2023. https://doi.org/10.1210/clinem/dgad373.
22. Mancini A, Howard SR, Marelli F, et al. LGR4 deficiency results in delayed puberty through impaired Wnt/beta-catenin signaling. JCI Insight 2020;5(11). https://doi.org/10.1172/jci.insight.133434.
23. Howard SR, Guasti L, Poliandri A, et al. Contributions of Function-Altering Variants in Genes Implicated in Pubertal Timing and Body Mass for Self-Limited Delayed Puberty. J Clin Endocrinol Metab 2018;103(2):649–59.
24. Vezzoli V, Hrvat F, Goggi G, et al. Genetic architecture of self-limited delayed puberty and congenital hypogonadotropic hypogonadism. Front Endocrinol 2022; 13:1069741.
25. Vazquez MJ, Velasco I, Tena-Sempere M. Novel mechanisms for the metabolic control of puberty: implications for pubertal alterations in early-onset obesity and malnutrition. J Endocrinol 2019;242(2):R51–65.
26. Barabas K, Szabo-Meleg E, Abraham IM. Effect of Inflammation on Female Gonadotropin-Releasing Hormone (GnRH) Neurons: Mechanisms and Consequences. Int J Mol Sci 2020;21(2). https://doi.org/10.3390/ijms21020529.
27. Cano Sokoloff N, Misra M, Ackerman KE. Exercise, Training, and the Hypothalamic-Pituitary-Gonadal Axis in Men and Women. Front Horm Res 2016;47:27–43.
28. Delaney A, Burkholder AB, Lavender CA, et al. Increased Burden of Rare Sequence Variants in GnRH-Associated Genes in Women With Hypothalamic Amenorrhea. J Clin Endocrinol Metab 2021;106(3):e1441–52.
29. Howard SR, Dunkel L. Delayed Puberty-Phenotypic Diversity, Molecular Genetic Mechanisms, and Recent Discoveries. Endocr Rev 2019;40(5):1285–317.
30. Gravholt CH, Andersen NH, Conway GS, et al. Clinical practice guidelines for the care of girls and women with Turner syndrome: proceedings from the 2016 Cincinnati International Turner Syndrome Meeting. Eur J Endocrinol 2017;177(3): G1–70.

31. Eskenazi S, Bachelot A, Hugon-Rodin J, et al. Next Generation Sequencing Should Be Proposed to Every Woman With "Idiopathic" Primary Ovarian Insufficiency. J Endocr Soc 2021;5(7):bvab032.
32. Aung Y, Kokotsis V, Yin KN, et al. Key features of puberty onset and progression can help distinguish self-limited delayed puberty from congenital hypogonadotrophic hypogonadism. Front Endocrinol 2023;14:1226839.
33. Reinehr T, Hoffmann E, Rothermel J, et al. Characteristic dynamics of height and weight in preschool boys with constitutional delay of growth and puberty or hypogonadotropic hypogonadism. Clin Endocrinol 2019;91(3):424–31.
34. Harrington J, Palmert MR. Clinical review: Distinguishing constitutional delay of growth and puberty from isolated hypogonadotropic hypogonadism: critical appraisal of available diagnostic tests. J Clin Endocrinol Metab 2012;97(9):3056–67.
35. Cavallo F, Mohn A, Chiarelli F, et al. Evaluation of Bone Age in Children: A Mini-Review. Front Pediatr 2021;9:580314.
36. Coutant R, Biette-Demeneix E, Bouvattier C, et al. Baseline inhibin B and anti-Mullerian hormone measurements for diagnosis of hypogonadotropic hypogonadism (HH) in boys with delayed puberty. J Clin Endocrinol Metab 2010; 95(12):5225–32.
37. Gao Y, Du Q, Liu L, et al. Serum inhibin B for differentiating between congenital hypogonadotropic hypogonadism and constitutional delay of growth and puberty: a systematic review and meta-analysis. Endocrine 2021;72(3):633–43.
38. Mosbah H, Bouvattier C, Maione L, et al. GnRH stimulation testing and serum inhibin B in males: insufficient specificity for discriminating between congenital hypogonadotropic hypogonadism from constitutional delay of growth and puberty. Hum Reprod 2020;35(10):2312–22.
39. Chaudhary S, Walia R, Bhansali A, et al. FSH-stimulated Inhibin B (FSH-iB): A Novel Marker for the Accurate Prediction of Pubertal Outcome in Delayed Puberty. J Clin Endocrinol Metab 2021;106(9):e3495–505.
40. Chan YM, Lippincott MF, Sales Barroso P, et al. Using Kisspeptin to Predict Pubertal Outcomes for Youth With Pubertal Delay. J Clin Endocrinol Metab 2020; 105(8):e2717–25.
41. Saengkaew T, Patel HR, Banerjee K, et al. Genetic evaluation supports differential diagnosis in adolescent patients with delayed puberty. Eur J Endocrinol 2021; 185(5):617–27.
42. Costa-Barbosa FA, Balasubramanian R, Keefe KW, et al. Prioritizing genetic testing in patients with Kallmann syndrome using clinical phenotypes. J Clin Endocrinol Metab 2013;98(5):E943–53.
43. Salonia A, Rastrelli G, Hackett G, et al. Paediatric and adult-onset male hypogonadism. Nat Rev Dis Primers 2019;5(1):38.
44. Klein KO, Phillips SA. Review of Hormone Replacement Therapy in Girls and Adolescents with Hypogonadism. J Pediatr Adolesc Gynecol 2019;32(5):460–8.
45. Jonsdottir-Lewis E, Feld A, Ciarlo R, et al. Timing of Pubertal Onset in Girls and Boys With Constitutional Delay. J Clin Endocrinol Metab 2021;106(9):e3693–703.
46. Gaysina D, Richards M, Kuh D, et al. Pubertal maturation and affective symptoms in adolescence and adulthood: Evidence from a prospective birth cohort. Dev Psychopathol 2015;27(4 Pt 1):1331–40.
47. Crowne EC, Shalet SM, Wallace WH, et al. Final height in boys with untreated constitutional delay in growth and puberty. Arch Dis Child 1990;65(10):1109–12.
48. Kariola L, Varimo T, Huopio H, et al. Health-related quality of life in boys with constitutional delay of growth and puberty. Front Endocrinol 2022;13:1028828.

49. Wehkalampi K, Vangonen K, Laine T, et al. Progressive reduction of relative height in childhood predicts adult stature below target height in boys with constitutional delay of growth and puberty. Horm Res 2007;68(2):99–104.
50. Wehkalampi K, Pakkila K, Laine T, et al. Adult height in girls with delayed pubertal growth. Horm Res Paediatr 2011;76(2):130–5.
51. Cools BL, Rooman R, Op De Beeck L, et al. Boys with a simple delayed puberty reach their target height. Horm Res 2008;70(4):209–14.
52. Osterbrand M, Fors H, Norjavaara E. Pharmacological treatment for pubertal progression in boys with delayed or slow progression of puberty: A small-scale randomized study with testosterone enanthate and testosterone undecanoate treatment. Front Endocrinol 2023;14:1158219.
53. Mastromattei S, Todisco T, Chioma L, et al. Efficacy of short-term induction therapy with low-dose testosterone as a diagnostic tool in the workup of delayed growth and puberty in boys. J Endocrinol Invest 2022;45(12):2377–84.
54. Dutta D, Singla R, Surana V, et al. Efficacy and Safety of Letrozole in the Management of Constitutional Delay in Growth and Puberty: A Systematic Review and Meta-analysis. J Clin Res Pediatr Endocrinol 2022;14(2):131–44.
55. Varimo T, Huopio H, Kariola L, et al. Letrozole versus testosterone for promotion of endogenous puberty in boys with constitutional delay of growth and puberty: a randomised controlled phase 3 trial. Lancet Child Adolesc Health 2019;3(2):109–20.
56. Wickman S, Sipila I, Ankarberg-Lindgren C, et al. A specific aromatase inhibitor and potential increase in adult height in boys with delayed puberty: a randomised controlled trial. Lancet 2001;357(9270):1743–8.

Hypogonadotropic Hypogonadism

Kanthi Bangalore Krishna, MD[a],*, John S. Fuqua, MD[b],
Selma F. Witchel, MD[a]

KEYWORDS

- Delayed puberty • Hypogonadotropic hypogonadism • Amenorrhea

KEY POINTS

- Delayed puberty is defined as absent testicular enlargement in boys or breast development in girls at an age that is 2 to 2.5 SDS later than the mean age at which these events occur in the population (traditionally, 14 years in boys and 13 years in girls).
- Hypogonadotropic hypogonadism (HH) can be classified into four major categories: congenital HH (CHH) with anosmia; CHH without anosmia; acquired/functional HH; and pituitary-dependent gonadotropin deficiency.
- The overarching goal of HH treatment in males is to mimic endogenous puberty in younger boys with known HH or to induce more rapid development of male secondary sex characteristics in older boys.
- With appropriate hormone replacement therapy, female patients with HH can develop secondary sexual characteristics, maintain normal sex steroid concentrations, and lead healthy sexual lives.
- With appropriate treatment, men and women with HH may be able to achieve fertility.

INTRODUCTION

Puberty consists of two components: gonadarche and adrenarche. Gonadarche reflects reactivation of the hypothalamic gonadotropin releasing hormone (GnRH) pulse generator, characterized by increased pulsatile secretion of GnRH from the hypothalamus. This promotes pulsatile pituitary gonadotropin secretion which, in turn, stimulates the growth and maturation of the gonads accompanied by increasing gonadal sex steroid secretion. Adrenarche refers to pubertal adrenal maturation, manifested by pubarche which is the development of pubic and axillary hair. As adrenarche is independent of gonadarche, its absence is excluded from the definition of delayed

[a] Division of Pediatric Endocrinology and Diabetes, UPMC Childrens Hospital of Pittsburgh, 4401 Penn Avenue, Pittsburgh, PA 15224, USA; [b] Division of Pediatric Endocrinology, Indiana University School of Medicine, 705 Riley Hospital Drive, Room 5960, Indianapolis, IN 46202, USA
* Corresponding author. UPMC Childrens Hospital of Pittsburgh, 4401 Penn Ave, Pittsburgh, PA 15224.
E-mail address: bangalorekrishnak2@upmc.edu

Endocrinol Metab Clin N Am 53 (2024) 279–292
https://doi.org/10.1016/j.ecl.2024.01.008

puberty. The age at onset of puberty may be associated with health consequences later in adulthood. As would be anticipated, later age at menarche is associated with increased risks for osteopenia and osteoporotic fractures in women, possibly due to shorter duration of estrogen exposure.[1]

Studies of twins have shown that the timing of puberty is highly heritable. Epidemiologic data suggest that approximately 50% to 75% of the variation in the age at onset of puberty is influenced by genetics.[2] Other factors such as nutrition, metabolism, environment, and general health can also influence the onset and tempo of puberty. Delayed puberty is traditionally defined as a lack of testicular enlargement $\geq$4 mL in boys or breast development in girls at an age that is 2 to 2.5 SD later than the mean age at which these events occur in the population (traditionally, 14 years in boys and 13 years in girls),[3] or based on puberty nomograms in some populations.[4] The lack of menarche by age 16 years or by 3 years post-thelarche is considered abnormal. Some children show initial pubertal maturation yet fail to complete puberty.[5]

One cause of delayed/absent puberty is hypogonadotropic hypogonadism (HH), which refers to inadequate hypothalamic/pituitary function leading to deficient production of sex steroids in males and females. Individuals with HH typically have normal gonads, and thus HH differs from hypergonadotropic hypogonadism, which is associated with primary gonadal insufficiency. HH may be congenital or acquired and is distinct from constitutional delay of growth and puberty (CDGP).[6] Although HH can rarely be transient or intermittent, CDGP is transient by definition and is considered to be a variant of normal development (see Jennifer Harrington's article, "Delayed Puberty Including Constitutional Delay: Differential and Outcome," in this issue). The exact incidence of HH is unclear, likely due to ascertainment bias and missed diagnosis. To understand the disorders leading to inadequate hypothalamic/pituitary function, a review of the development of the GnRH neuronal system and components of the hypothalamic pituitary gonadal axis (HPG) axis is germane as discussed in the following.

ONTOGENY OF GnRH NEURONS

Reproductive competence depends on the proper development of the GnRH neuron system. In the human fetus, GnRH neurons initially develop in the olfactory placode outside the central nervous system. Subsequently, accompanied by olfactory-derived axons, olfactory epithelial sheath cells, and blood vessels, the GnRH neurons migrate toward the cribriform plate. Migration of the GnRH neurons seems to pause at the nasal/forebrain junction before crossing the cribriform plate. During this "pause" phase, multiple tissues, chemokines, growth factors, and neurotransmitters seem to form gradients influencing movement of GnRH neurons. On reaching the hypothalamus, the GnRH neurons disperse to their final locations, sending projections to the median eminence.[7]

The precise origin and specific factors responsible for the specification, differentiation, connectivity, and stabilization of GnRH neurons remain enigmatic.[8]

COMPONENTS OF THE HPG AXIS

The human hypothalamus contains approximately 2000 diffusely distributed GnRH neurons. The mammalian GnRH neuron displays unique characteristics.[9] At the median eminence, their dendritic fibers are intertwined, encased by tanycytes (specialized ependymal cells of the third ventricle), project to blood vessels, and receive synaptic inputs.[10] At the median eminence, the GnRH neurons intermittently discharge GnRH into the primary plexus of the hypophysial portal circulation, stimulating pulsatile leutinizing hormone (LH) and follicle stimulating hormone (FSH) secretion. Generally, GnRH pulses correspond 1:1 with LH pulses.

The GnRH neurons are physically located within a neuronal network secreting three neuropeptides: kisspeptin, neurokinin B, and dynorphin. These neurons, labeled the kisspeptin-neurokinin B-dynorphin (KNDy) neurons, are in close proximity to glial cells such as tanycytes, astrocytes, and ependymal cells. The KNDy neurons in the infundibular nucleus of the hypothalamus seem to comprise the major elements of the GnRH pulse generator, with kisspeptin and neurokinin B partaking in major facets of GnRH secretion.

Gonadotropin-releasing hormone is a decapeptide (pGlu-His-Trp-Ser-Trp-Gly-Leu-Arg-Pro-Gly-NH$_2$) derived from a 92-amino acid precursor, prepro-GnRH, originally characterized in 1984.[11] LH and FSH are synthesized in the same gonadotroph cells in the anterior pituitary. LH and FSH are glycoproteins with identical alpha subunits and distinct beta subunits that confer hormone specificity. Glycosylation seems to influence hormone stability, circulating serum half-life, protein folding, cellular trafficking, and receptor signaling. The patterns of gonadotropin secretion prenatally and postnatally and their relationships to the gonadal steroids, testosterone and estradiol, have been well characterized. In adult men, pulse frequency is relatively constant at approximately one pulse every 90 to 120 minutes. Among women, pulse frequency varies across the menstrual cycle from approximately one pulse per hour during the follicular phase and one pulse every 180 minutes during the luteal phase.[12] The actions of LH and FSH are mediated by their cognate seven-transmembrane domain G protein-coupled receptors, the luteinizing hormone/choriogonadotropin receptor (LHCGR) and FSH receptor, respectively.

Reproduction is metabolically costly, requiring ample energy reserve to support the onset of puberty and maintenance of fertility. Energy reserves are signaled in part by leptin release from adipose tissue. Patients with leptin deficiency manifest delayed puberty that resolves with leptin treatment.[13] Although initially conceptualized as the proximate factor initiating puberty, leptin functions as an obligatory permissive factor for pubertal development that informs the hypothalamus of overall energy status. Much remains to be discovered about how the hypothalamic network monitors energy balance and transmits information to the GnRH pulse generator to influence kisspeptin secretion.[14]

CLASSIFICATION OF HYPOGONADOTROPIC HYPOGONADISM

HH can be classified into four major categories: (1) congenital HH (CHH) with anosmia; (2) CHH without anosmia; (3) acquired/functional HH; and (4) pituitary-dependent gonadotropin deficiency. However, it has become apparent that phenotypic heterogeneity exists for anosmia; the extent of anosmia can vary among family members within a single family. Additional subclassifications include genetic, anatomic, or functional. Self-limited delayed puberty, also known as constitutional delay, is discussed in Jennifer Harrington's article, "Delayed Puberty Including Constitutional Delay: Differential and Outcome," in this issue.

CONGENITAL HYPOGONADOTROPIC HYPOGONADISM

In many instances, CHH is due to deficient production, secretion, or action of gonadotropin-releasing hormone (GnRH) and is characterized by incomplete or absent puberty in the setting of low gonadotropin and sex steroid concentrations. Given the developmental origins of GnRH neurons in the olfactory placode, CHH may be associated with anosmia (absent sense of smell) or hyposmia (reduced sense of smell). This association is known as Kallmann syndrome. CHH can present as isolated congenital GnRH deficiency or can be syndromic. Syndromic CHH is associated with other developmental anomalies (**Table 1**). In some instances, HH may be associated with additional anterior pituitary hormone deficiencies.

Prenatal testicular testosterone secretion is crucial for the development of the external genital structures in boys. Boys with CHH may present with micropenis because fetal penile growth typically occurs after the 12th week of gestation when external genital differentiation has been completed. In other words, boys with CHH generally do not have otherwise atypical external genitalia. The explanation for this finding is that human chorionic gonadotropin (hCG) drives fetal testicular testosterone secretion early during gestation when the initial development of the external genitalia occurs. The pituitary gland begins to secrete gonadotropins during the second trimester, with LH and FSH becoming detectable in fetal blood after 14 weeks of gestation.

Genetics of Hypogonadotropic Hypogonadism

The recognition that HH was associated with deleterious GnRH receptor variants fueled the ongoing pursuit to identify genes associated with altered HPG function.[15] Inheritance patterns include autosomal dominant, autosomal recessive, X-linked, and oligogenic. An oligogenic pattern refers to the presence of concomitant variants in several different genes, leading to a CHH phenotype. To date, more than 50 such genes have been identified. Genome-wide association studies continue to expand knowledge regarding genes associated with CHH (**Fig. 1**). These genes may be classified as being associated with anosmia/hyposmia (Kallmann syndrome) or normosmia (**Table 2**). The classic example of anosmic CHH is X-linked Kallmann syndrome due to anosmin-1 (*ANOS1*) variants. The absence of this protein prevents migration of GnRH neurons to the hypothalamus. Additional features of *ANOS1* mutations include unilateral renal agenesis, sensorineural hearing loss, dental agenesis, synkinesia (alternating mirror movements), and cleft lip/palate.

Some genetic variants have additional findings. Defects in *NROB1* encoding the DAX1 protein are associated with CHH and congenital adrenal hypoplasia. The

Table 1	
Syndromic causes of congenital hypogonadotropic hypogonadism	
Gene	**Syndrome**
Several genes including *HESX1*, *PROP1*, *LHX3*, and *LHX4*	Septo-optic dysplasia/panhypopituitarism
Loss of paternal 15q11.2	Prader–Willi syndrome
CHD7	CHARGE syndrome
Several genes including *BBS1*, *BBS10*, *BBS2*, *BBS9*, *MKKS*, *BBS12*, *MKS1*, *BBS4*, *BBS7*, and *TTC8*	Bardet–Biedl syndrome
SOX10	Waardenburg syndrome
OTUD4, *PNPLA6*, *RNF216*, *STUB1*	Gordon Holmes syndrome
HFE	HFE-associated hereditary hemochromatosis
TUBB3	TUBB3 E410 K syndrome
RAB3GAP1, *RAB3GAP2*, *RAB18*, *TBC1D20*	Warburg micro syndrome/Martsolf syndrome
Xp21 microdeletion encompassing NROB1 (DAX1) and DMD	Xp21 deletion syndrome
Xp22.3 microdeletion encompassing ANOS1	Xp22.3 deletion syndrome
IGSF1	X-linked with central hypothyroidism, macroorchidism

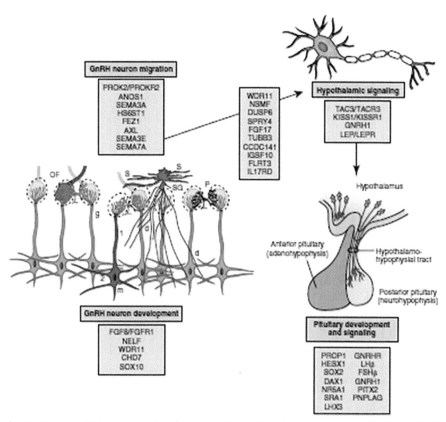

Fig. 1. Genes in GnRH neuron development. Illustration showing genes and roles in GnRH neuron and pituitary development. (Reprinted with permission: Oberfield SE, Witchel SF. In Strauss JF, Barbieri RL, Dokras A, Williams CJ, Williams SZ, eds. Yen and Jaffe's Reproductive Endocrinology, 9th ed. Elsevier, Philadelphia, 2023.)

CHARGE syndrome, characterized by coloboma, heart anomalies, choanal atresia, growth retardation, and genital and ear anomalies, is due to variants in *CHD7* that may lead to isolated CHH or CHH associated with other clinical features.

PITUITARY HORMONE DEFICIENCY

Gonadotropin deficiency can occur in patients with combined pituitary hormone deficiency (CPHD). Some patients also have septo-optic dysplasia. Typically, genetic variants associated with CPHD are involved in development of the head or pituitary gland development. Specific genes associated with CPHD include *LHX4*, *HESX1*, *PITX3*, *GATA2*, *PROP1*, and *SOX2*. Detailed discussion of these genes can be found elsewhere.[16] Inactivating variants of the specific β-subunits of LH and FSH have been described.[17] Ig superfamily member 1 (IGSF1) deficiency is an X-linked disorder associated with central hypothyroidism, macroorchidism, and delayed puberty.[18]

ACQUIRED HYPOGONADISM

Acquired HH reflects central nervous system (CNS) dysfunction associated with trauma, tumor, infection, or another intracranial processes (**Box 1**). Craniopharyngiomas and

Table 2
Inheritance pattern of genes associated with congenital hypogonadotropic hypogonadism

Gene	Product	Olfactory Function	Inheritance Pattern
ANOS1/KAL1	Anosmin-1	Anosmic	X-linked
SEMA3A	Semaphorin 3A	Anosmic	AD with variable expression
SOX10	Sex-determining region Y-Box 10 transcription factor	Anosmic	AD with variable expression
IL17RD	Interleukin-17 receptor D	Anosmic	AD with variable expression/AR
FEZF1	FEZ family zinc finger 1	Anosmic	AR
FGFR1	Fibroblast growth factor receptor 1	Anosmic or normosmic	AD with variable expression
FGF8	Fibroblast growth factor 8	Anosmic or normosmic	AD with variable expression
KLB	β-Klotho	Anosmic or normosmic	AD with variable expression
PROK2 and PROKR2	Prokineticin 2 and its receptor	Anosmic or normosmic	AR/oligogenic
CHD7	Chromodomain helicase DNA-binding protein 7	Anosmic or normosmic	AD with variable expression
NSMF	N-methyl-D-aspartate receptor synaptonuclear signaling and neuronal migration factor	Anosmic or normosmic	Oligogenic
HS6ST1	Heparin sulfate 6-o-sulfotransferase 1	Anosmic or normosmic	Autosomal dominant/oligogenic
FGF17	Fibroblast growth factor 17	Anosmic or normosmic	Autosomal dominant/oligogenic
SPRY4	Sprouty homolog 4	Anosmic or normosmic	Autosomal dominant/oligogenic
DUSP6	Dual specificity phosphatase 6/MKP3-mitogen-activated protein kinase phosphatase	Anosmic or normosmic	Autosomal dominant/oligogenic
FLRT3	Fibronectin leucine rich transmembrane protein 3	Anosmic or normosmic	Indeterminate/oligogenic
WDR11	WD repeat-containing protein 11	Anosmic or normosmic	Indeterminate/oligogenic
AXL	AXL receptor tyrosine kinase	Anosmic or normosmic	Indeterminate/oligogenic
GNRHR	GnRH receptor	Normosmic	Autosomal recessive
GNRH1	Prepro-GnRH	Normosmic	Autosomal recessive
KISS1R	Kisspeptin receptor 1	Normosmic	Autosomal recessive
KISS1	Kisspeptin	Normosmic	Autosomal recessive
TAC3	Neurokinin B	Normosmic	Autosomal recessive
TAC3R	Neurokinin B receptor	Normosmic	Autosomal recessive

Box 1
Causes of acquired secondary hypogonadism
Intracranial space-occupying lesions (eg, tumors/cysts)
Infiltrative disease (eg, histiocytosis, sarcoidosis, or hemochromatosis)
Infection (eg, meningitis)
Pituitary apoplexy (bleeding into pituitary gland)
Pituitary adenoma
Rathke's cleft cyst
CNS trauma
CNS irradiation
Chemotherapy
Chronic disease (eg, diabetes, anorexia, obesity, and chronic kidney disease)
Excessive exercise
Critical illness
Chronic opioid, glucocorticoid, or anabolic steroid use
Hyperprolactinemia, prolonged hypothyroidism

germ cell tumors can disrupt the hypothalamic–pituitary stalk or directly impact pituitary function to inhibit gonadotropin production. Intracranial surgeries and/or cranial radiation therapy greater than 30 Gy are known risk factors for HH. Moderate to severe trauma to the brain can induce hypothalamic–pituitary dysfunction. Inflammatory, autoimmune, and infiltrative diseases of the pituitary gland are rare causes of acquired HH. Curiously, hemochromatosis preferentially affects gonadotrophs resulting in isolated HH.

FUNCTIONAL

Functional HH reflects the hypothalamic response to intense physical activities, intense emotional stress, nutrition–caloric deficiency, or chronic systemic illness.[19] Chronic systemic illnesses associated with delayed or arrested puberty include inflammatory bowel disease, cystic fibrosis, sickle cell anemia, thalassemia, hypothyroidism, restrictive eating disorder, and poorly controlled type 1 diabetes mellitus, among others. Typically, effective treatment of the underlying disorder is associated with pubertal progression and reversibility of the functional HH.

Peripheral signals such as leptin convey information about nutritional status to indirectly modulate GnRH neurosecretion. Indeed, the reproductive phenotype of inactivating variants involving leptin or its receptor emphasizes the importance of adequate nutritional status for HPG axis function.

Acquired HH can also be caused by drugs, infiltrative or infectious pituitary lesions, hyperprolactinemia, brain trauma, pituitary/brain radiation, and systemic diseases such as hemochromatosis, sarcoidosis, or histiocytosis.

DIAGNOSIS OF HYPOGONADOTROPIC HYPOGONADISM

CHH may be diagnosed in males as cryptorchidism with or without micropenis during the mini-puberty of infancy (a period of transient re-activation of the HPG axis) or in adolescence when patients fail to develop pubertal changes. HH is typically a diagnosis of exclusion after confirming the absence of structural changes or acquired conditions. For some children with syndromic HH, accompanying signs and symptoms often point to HH. If the adolescent presents with any neurologic symptoms (eg, headache, visual disturbances, recurrent emesis) or signs (eg, focal deficits, visual field defects), brain imaging must be completed.

Distinguishing HH from constitutional delay may be challenging. Some patients with HH participate in a diagnostic odyssey involving multiple health care providers and medical testing. Further, the traditional approach of "watchful waiting" may hinder the diagnostic process and negatively impact psychosocial health. Like those with other rare disorders, individuals with CHH may feel different and isolated from peers. Speculation regarding potential infertility/subfertility may elicit added distress for the patient and extended family.[20] Genetic testing has become increasingly available and may be helpful because the genetic architecture differs between HH and CDGP.[21]

TREATMENT OF HYPOGONADOTROPIC HYPOGONADISM IN MALES

The overarching goal of HH treatment is to mimic endogenous puberty in younger boys with known HH or to induce more rapid development of male secondary sex characteristics in older boys. Induction of normal age-appropriate body composition, bone density, and psychosocial functioning are other important goals.

Timing of Treatment

In some cases, HH is detected early in life because of small phallic size and an absent mini-puberty of infancy. When it is certain that spontaneous puberty will not occur, the timing of pubertal induction should generally match the boy's peers or family history. More commonly, HH is not confirmed in infancy but may be possible based on patients' underlying diagnoses or treatments. In these cases, because there is no accepted diagnostic test for HH in peripubertal boys, watchful waiting is the first-line approach to exclude a simple delay in puberty. If testicular enlargement has not occurred by an arbitrary age, usually 14 years, there is a higher suspicion of HH, and treatment should begin. In older boys with acquired HH who have already begun puberty, treatment can commence once the diagnosis is confirmed.

Approaches to Treatment

Testosterone esters
Historically, treatment of HH in both early and later adolescence has been with injectable testosterone esters, usually testosterone cypionate, enanthate, or propionate. These preparations have a long track record of safety and efficacy and are inexpensive and easy to administer. Injectable testosterone reliably increases secondary sex characteristics such as penile enlargement, development of male-typical facial and body hair, linear growth, weight gain, deepening of the voice, and increased muscularity. However, it does not change testicular volume, which depends on gonadotropin secretion, particularly FSH. Similarly, it does not promote spermatogenesis, which requires both gonadotropins and high intra-testicular testosterone concentrations.[22] In addition, serum testosterone concentrations are elevated for several days after each injection but may reach subnormal trough levels before the next injection.

There are many other testosterone preparations available[23] that have been developed for use in adult men. Transdermal testosterone gels have become popular and avoid the need for injections and permit more stable testosterone concentrations. However, they require daily use and carry a risk for inadvertent transfer of testosterone to children and women. Oral testosterone undecanoate has been used for short-term treatment of constitutional delay of growth but is not yet generally recommended for pubertal induction in HH.[24] Testosterone esters may be injected subcutaneously, which decreases injection pain and maintains satisfactory pharmacokinetics.[25]

Several testosterone regimens have been proposed.[23] A common approach is a starting dose of injectable testosterone cypionate or enanthate of 50 mg monthly, increasing by 50 mg every 6 months to attain an adult dose of 150 to 250 mg every 2 to 4 weeks. Transdermal testosterone gel can be started at 10 mg of delivered testosterone every other day, with gradual increases over 2 to 3 years to reach an adult dose of 40 to 80 mg of delivered testosterone every day. Responsiveness varies, and some patients may require faster or slower advances. After reaching adult doses, serum testosterone levels may be monitored periodically. This may be done midway between injectable testosterone doses or before a dose as a trough level. In patients using transdermal testosterone gel, serum levels can be monitored at any time, as concentrations are stable over the course of the day.[26]

Gonadotropins

An alternative approach that is gaining popularity is the use of injectable gonadotropins to induce testicular maturation and growth, with the aim of promoting both endogenous testosterone secretion and Sertoli cell growth. This approach has been shown to stimulate spermatogenesis and increase the long-term chance of fertility.[27] Testicular growth may also confer psychological benefit for the patient. hCG, which stimulates the LH receptor, has been used alone or with recombinant FSH (rFSH) for this purpose.[23,28] In patients with known HH, gonadotropin therapy can be used until testicular growth and physical maturation have occurred, and the regimen can then be changed to testosterone for long-term maintenance. The collection of a semen sample at the completion of combination therapy can be considered.

Fertility in men with congenital hypogonadotropic hypogonadism: Use of gonadotropins

Many regimens have been published for gonadotropin stimulation that vary by the order of administration and the doses used. Many regimens call for a period of FSH treatment lasting for 1 to 12 months, following which hCG is added for 6 to 24 months to induce endogenous testosterone secretion and subsequent virilization.[23] This initial treatment with rFSH alone is predicted to lead to better Sertoli cell and testicular growth than hCG alone or combined with rFSH because testosterone exposure, either by direct testosterone administration or by hCG stimulation, may cause premature cessation of Sertoli cell proliferation.[29] Although gonadotropin treatment has advantages over testosterone treatment, it is burdensome for patients, requiring multiple injections weekly, and it may be difficult for some teens to complete. Similar regimens replicating endocrine regulation of spermatogenesis or exogenous gonadotropins may be used to induce fertility in adult men following initial testosterone treatment.[30] However, treatment tends to be more successful in men with acquired HH than those with CHH.[29]

Adverse Effects of Testosterone Treatment

Testosterone treatment in adolescent boys is generally safe. Gynecomastia is common in the untreated HH population, but testosterone administration may increase the incidence due to aromatization of testosterone to estradiol. Priapism occurs rarely in boys receiving testosterone. Dose-related increases in hematocrit are common, and routine monitoring of this is recommended after adult testosterone doses are reached.[31] Behavioral problems may arise but are usually manageable in neurotypical individuals. Adverse behaviors may require dose reduction, especially in those with neurocognitive disabilities.

TREATMENT OF HYPOGONADOTROPIC HYPOGONADISM IN FEMALES

With appropriate hormone replacement therapy, female patients with HH can develop secondary sexual characteristics, maintain normal sex steroid concentrations, lead healthy sexual lives, and may also achieve fertility.[32] Several regimens of treatment with different administration routes exist. The choice of treatment depends on the therapeutic goal, the timing of treatment, and the personal preference of each patient.[3] It is important to know that randomized controlled trials of hormonal treatment in HH and data from clinical observational studies are limited. There is no uniform treatment regimen used internationally.

In girls, the therapeutic objectives are breast development, uterine growth, cornification of the vaginal mucosa, feminine appearance, and promotion of psychosexual development with respect to emotional life and sexuality. In addition, pubertal induction also increases uterine size, which is important for future pregnancy. Finally, optimizing linear growth to achieve an adult height close to the target height range is important, along with acquiring normal bone mineral density. Most therapeutic regimens inducing feminization in CHH are not evidence-based and usually arise from expert opinions. Many regimens have mirrored Turner syndrome treatment.[33]

Approaches to Treatment

Estrogen preparations

Both oral and transdermal estradiol induce feminization; however, the available protocols vary widely.[34] Transdermal estradiol administration is often started at low doses, sometime just with nocturnal applications, with the goal of mimicking estradiol levels during early puberty. The estradiol dose should then be increased gradually every 4 to 6 months.[35] After maximizing breast development and/or after breakthrough bleeding, cyclic progesterone therapy is added. Thus, cyclic progesterone may be implemented 12 to 24 months after initiation of estrogen treatment. In most females with HH, this therapy is effective to induce breast development, promote normal secondary sex characteristics, increase uterine size, accelerate linear growth, and induce withdrawal bleeding. However, this treatment does not restore ovulation. Hormonal treatment is required in adult females with HH to maintain bone health, improve emotional and sexual life, and promote general well-being.[33]

Treatment of functional hypothalamic amenorrhea (HA) involves nutritional rehabilitation as well as reductions in stress and exercise levels.[36] Many women with functional HA have an element of disordered eating or an incipient eating disorder that may require psychological support to facilitate a change in eating habits. In those with a formally diagnosed eating disorder, such as anorexia nervosa or bulimia nervosa, referral to a specialized eating disorder service is recommended to enable these patients to be appropriately treated by a multidisciplinary team, including psychiatrists. Improving the energy deficit often requires behavioral changes, and weight gain may need to be supervised by a registered dietitian or nutritionist. Reversing the negative energy balance by restoration of body weight or fat mass and/or reduction in exercise intensity may be sufficient to restore menses and improve rates of conception in some patients with functional HA. Some clinical trials have demonstrated the potential efficacy of leptin treatment in functional HA.[37] Hormone replacement therapy should be considered if this alone fails to restore menses and/there are ongoing skeletal or psychosocial concerns.

Fertility in women with congenital hypogonadotropic hypogonadism: Use of gonadotropins

Infertility in women with CHH is caused by impaired pituitary secretion of gonadotropins, leading to impaired ovarian stimulation and chronic anovulation. The combination of small ovaries, decreased antral follicle count, and low circulating anti-Müllerian hormone concentrations observed in women with CHH could suggest an alteration in ovarian reserve and a poor fertility prognosis. However, ovulation induction can still lead to a good fertility outcome.[38] Before considering ovulation induction, radiographic studies to evaluate both the integrity and the permeability of the uterine cavity and fallopian tubes should be completed. The goal of ovulation induction therapy in female patients with CHH is to obtain a mono-ovulation to avoid multiple pregnancies. Ovulation can be achieved either with pulsatile GnRH therapy or stimulation with gonadotropins: either extracted or rFSH treatment followed by hCG or human recombinant LH (rLH) to trigger ovulation.[39,40] The therapeutic choice will depend on the expertise of each center and the local availability of the different medical therapeutics.[38] Estradiol is necessary to maintain optimal cervical mucus production and endometrial thickness, which in turn are needed for sperm transit and embryo implantation. Typically, subcutaneous human menopausal gonadotropins (hMGs; FSH plus hCG) are sufficient to induce ovulation and the starting dose of hMG is often increased or decreased depending on the ovarian response as assessed by repeated serum estradiol measurements or by using ultrasonography to count and measure maturing follicles every other day.[41]

SUMMARY

HH refers to a broad group of disorders characterized by impaired neuroendocrine function resulting in delayed puberty. Because the identification of the GnRH receptor genetic variant associated with CHH, knowledge regarding inheritance patterns and specific genes has greatly expanded. The use of focused genetic panels has hastened the diagnostic process by facilitating molecular diagnosis. Nevertheless, the number of genes included on the test panels is limited, which means that "negative results" cannot exclude the diagnosis of CHH. Another caveat is that increasing numbers of "variants of unknown significance" are detected. Hence, distinguishing novel rare deleterious variants from benign variants may be problematic in some situations.

CLINICS CARE POINTS

- Delayed puberty is defined by the absence of breast development by age 13 years in girls or absence of testicular enlargement $\geq$ 4 mL by age 14 years in boys.

- Congenital hypogonadotropic hypogonadism is due to deficient production, secretion, or action of GnRH and is characterized by incomplete or absent puberty in the setting of low gonadotropin and sex steroid concentrations.

- In some cases, hypogonadotropic hypogonadism (HH) is detected early in life because of small phallic size and an absent mini-puberty of infancy. When it is certain that spontaneous puberty will not occur, the timing of pubertal induction should generally match the boy's peers or family history.

- The choice of HH treatment depends on the therapeutic goal, the timing of treatment, and the personal preference of each patient.

DISCLOSURE

The authors have nothing to disclose.

REFERENCES

1. Naves M, Díaz-López JB, Gómez C, et al. Determinants of incidence of osteoporotic fractures in the female Spanish population older than 50. Osteoporosis Int 2005;16(12):2013–7.
2. Saengkaew T, Howard SR. Genetics of pubertal delay. Clin Endocrinol 2022; 97(4):473–82.
3. Palmert MR, Dunkel L. Clinical practice. Delayed puberty. N Engl J Med 2012; 366(5):443–53.
4. Rodanaki M, Rask E, Lodefalk M. Delayed puberty in boys in central Sweden: an observational study on diagnosing and management in clinical practice. BMJ Open 2022;12(2):e057088.
5. Howard SRQR. Outcomes and experiences of adults with congenital hypogonadism can inform improvements in the management of delayed puberty. J Pediatr Endocrinol Metab. Nov 2023;37(1):1–7.
6. Aung Y, Kokotsis V, Yin KN, et al. Key features of puberty onset and progression can help distinguish self-limited delayed puberty from congenital hypogonadotrophic hypogonadism. Front Endocrinol 2023;14:1226839.
7. Duittoz AH, Forni PE, Giacobini P, et al. Development of the gonadotropin-releasing hormone system. J Neuroendocrinol 2022;34(5):e13087.
8. Chung WC, Tsai PS. The initiation and maintenance of gonadotropin-releasing hormone neuron identity in congenital hypogonadotropic hypogonadism. Front Endocrinol 2023;14.
9. Herbison AE. Control of puberty onset and fertility by gonadotropin-releasing hormone neurons. Nat Rev Endocrinol 2016;12(8):452–66.
10. Wang L, Guo W, Shen X, et al. Different dendritic domains of the GnRH neuron underlie the pulse and surge modes of GnRH secretion in female mice. Elife 2020;9.
11. Hayflick JS, Adelman JP, Seeburg PH. The Complete Nucleotide-Sequence of the Human Gonadotropin-Releasing Hormone Gene. Nucleic Acids Res 1989;17(15): 6403–4.
12. Reame N, Sauder SE, Kelch RP, et al. Pulsatile Gonadotropin-Secretion during the Human Menstrual-Cycle - Evidence for Altered Frequency of Gonadotropin-Releasing Hormone-Secretion. J Clin Endocr Metab 1984;59(2):328–37.
13. Farooqi IS, Jebb SA, Langmack G, et al. Effects of recombinant leptin therapy in a child with congenital leptin deficiency. N Engl J Med 1999;341(12):879–84.
14. Navarro VM. Metabolic regulation of kisspeptin - the link between energy balance and reproduction. Nat Rev Endocrinol 2020;16(8):407–20.
15. de Roux N, Young J, Misrahi M, et al. A family with hypogonadotropic hypogonadism and mutations in the gonadotropin-releasing hormone receptor. N Engl J Med 1997;337(22):1597–602.
16. Fang Q, George AS, Brinkmeier ML, et al. Genetics of Combined Pituitary Hormone Deficiency: Roadmap into the Genome Era. Endocr Rev 2016;37(6): 636–75.
17. Cangiano B, Swee D, Quinton R, et al. Genetics of congenital hypogonadotropic hypogonadism: peculiarities and phenotype of an oligogenic disease. Hum Genet 2021;140(1):77–111.

18. Joustra SD, Heinen CA, Schoenmakers N, et al. IGSF1 Deficiency: Lessons From an Extensive Case Series and Recommendations for Clinical Management. J Clin Endocr Metab 2016;101(4):1627–36.
19. Esquivel-Zuniga R, Rogol AD. Functional hypogonadism in adolescence: an overlooked cause of secondary hypogonadism. Endocr Connect 2023;12(11).
20. Dwyer AA, Smith N, Quinton R. Psychological Aspects of Congenital Hypogonadotropic Hypogonadism. Front Endocrinol 2019;10:353.
21. Cassatella D, Howard SR, Acierno JS, et al. Congenital hypogonadotropic hypogonadism and constitutional delay of growth and puberty have distinct genetic architectures. Eur J Endocrinol 2018;178(4):377–88.
22. Smith LB, Walker WH. The regulation of spermatogenesis by androgens. Semin Cell Dev Biol 2014;30:2–13.
23. Nordenstrom A, Ahmed SF, van den Akker E, et al. Pubertal induction and transition to adult sex hormone replacement in patients with congenital pituitary or gonadal reproductive hormone deficiency: an Endo-ERN clinical practice guideline. Eur J Endocrinol 2022;186(6):G9–49.
24. Federici S, Goggi G, Quinton R, et al. New and Consolidated Therapeutic Options for Pubertal Induction in Hypogonadism: In-depth Review of the Literature. Endocr Rev 2022;43(5):824–51.
25. Figueiredo MG, Gagliano-Juca T, Basaria S. Testosterone Therapy With Subcutaneous Injections: A Safe, Practical, and Reasonable Option. J Clin Endocrinol Metab 2022;107(3):614–26.
26. Wang C, Berman N, Longstreth JA, et al. Pharmacokinetics of transdermal testosterone gel in hypogonadal men: application of gel at one site versus four sites: a General Clinical Research Center Study. J Clin Endocrinol Metab 2000;85(3):964–9.
27. Rohayem J, Hauffa BP, Zacharin M, et al. Testicular growth and spermatogenesis: new goals for pubertal hormone replacement in boys with hypogonadotropic hypogonadism? -a multicentre prospective study of hCG/rFSH treatment outcomes during adolescence. Clin Endocrinol 2017;86(1):75–87.
28. Young J, Xu C, Papadakis GE, et al. Clinical Management of Congenital Hypogonadotropic Hypogonadism. Endocr Rev 2019;40(2):669–710.
29. Swee DS, Quinton R. Managing congenital hypogonadotrophic hypogonadism: a contemporary approach directed at optimizing fertility and long-term outcomes in males. Ther Adv Endocrinol Metab 2019;10. 2042018819826889.
30. Bouloux P, Warne DW, Loumaye E, et al. Efficacy and safety of recombinant human follicle-stimulating hormone in men with isolated hypogonadotropic hypogonadism. Fertil Steril 2002;77(2):270–3.
31. Stancampiano MR, Lucas-Herald AK, Russo G, et al. Testosterone Therapy in Adolescent Boys: The Need for a Structured Approach. Horm Res Paediatr 2019;92(4):215–28.
32. Kiess W, Conway G, Ritzen M, et al. Induction of puberty in the hypogonadal girl–practices and attitudes of pediatric endocrinologists in Europe. Horm Res 2002;57(1–2):66–71.
33. Klein KO, Phillips SA. Review of Hormone Replacement Therapy in Girls and Adolescents with Hypogonadism. J Pediatr Adolesc Gynecol 2019;32(5):460–8.
34. Ankarberg-Lindgren C, Kristrom B, Norjavaara E. Physiological estrogen replacement therapy for puberty induction in girls: a clinical observational study. Horm Res Paediatr 2014;81(4):239–44.
35. Harrington J, Palmert MR. An Approach to the Patient With Delayed Puberty. J Clin Endocrinol Metab 2022;107(6):1739–50.

36. Gordon CM, Ackerman KE, Berga SL, et al. Functional Hypothalamic Amenorrhea: An Endocrine Society Clinical Practice Guideline. J Clin Endocrinol Metab 2017;102(5):1413–39.
37. Chou SH, Chamberland JP, Liu X, et al. Leptin is an effective treatment for hypothalamic amenorrhea. Proc Natl Acad Sci U S A 2011;108(16):6585–90.
38. Abdelaal AE, Behery MA, Abdelkawi AF. Reproductive outcomes in women with hypogonadotrophic hypogonadism, a case series study. Middle East Fertil S 2021;26(1).
39. Guner JZ, Monsivais D, Yu HY, et al. Oral follicle-stimulating hormone receptor agonist affects granulosa cells differently than recombinant human FSH. Fertil Steril 2023;120(5):1061–70.
40. Martini AE, Beall S, Ball GD, et al. Fine-tuning the dose of recombinant human follicle-stimulating hormone alfa to individualize treatment in ovulation induction and ovarian stimulation cycles: a real-world database analysis. Front Endocrinol 2023;14.
41. Kaufmann R, Dunn R, Vaughn T, et al. Recombinant human luteinizing hormone, lutropin alfa, for the induction of follicular development and pregnancy in profoundly gonadotrophin-deficient women. Clin Endocrinol 2007;67(4):563–9.

Primary Amenorrhea and Premature Ovarian Insufficiency

Svetlana A. Yatsenko, MD[a,b], Selma F. Witchel, MD[c,*],
Catherine M. Gordon, MD, MS[d]

KEYWORDS

- Premature ovarian insufficiency • Turner syndrome • Differences in sex development
- Cancer survivorship • Low bone density • Estrogen deficiency
- Fertility preservation

KEY POINTS

- Premature ovarian insufficiency (POI) is defined as the lack of menses for at least 4 months associated with elevated serum follicle stimulating hormone and low estradiol concentrations obtained twice at least 1 month apart before the age of 40 years.
- A diagnostic quest or odyssey in pursuit of a cause that delays the diagnosis and frustrates the patient and her family should be avoided.
- Shared decision-making regarding the initiation of estradiol hormone replacement therapy.
- Assess for additional clinical features as appropriate, that is, cardiac echocardiology and renal ultrasound in girls diagnosed with Turner syndrome.

INTRODUCTION

Pubertal development in girls ranges between ages 8 and 13 years reflecting inter-individual variations attributed to ethnic, genetic, nutritional, and environmental elements. Typically, the first physical manifestation of puberty is breast development followed by menarche within 2 to 3 years.[1]

The ovary develops from the bipotential adrenogonadal primordium at ~28 days postconception. Precise spatiotemporal coordination of numerous factors promotes

[a] Department of Pathology, University of Pittsburgh, Magee-Womens Research Institute, Pittsburgh, PA, USA; [b] Department of Obstetrics, Gynecology and Reproductive Sciences, University of Pittsburgh, Magee-Womens Research Institute, Pittsburgh, PA, USA; [c] Division of Pediatric Endocrinology, Department of Pediatrics, UPMC Children's Hospital, University of Pittsburgh, Pittsburgh, PA, USA; [d] USDA/ARS Children's Nutrition Research Center, Baylor College of Medicine, Houston, TX, USA
* Corresponding author. Division of Pediatric Endocrinology, Department of Pediatrics, UPMC Children's Hospital, University of Pittsburgh, 4401 Penn Avenue, Pittsburgh, PA 15224.
E-mail address: witchelsf@upmc.edu

Endocrinol Metab Clin N Am 53 (2024) 293–305
https://doi.org/10.1016/j.ecl.2024.01.009   endo.theclinics.com

ovarian differentiation followed by the development of female internal and external genital structures. Primordial germ cells migrate to the developing ovary from the hindgut and form follicles, surrounded by somatic cells. At birth, ovaries contain approximately 1 to 2 million dormant primordial follicles. In neonates, the hypothalamic-pituitary-gonadal axis is transiently active as evident by gonadotropin and estradiol secretion during the first few months of life.[2] Ovaries then remain quiescent until the reactivation of the hypothalamic gonadotropin-releasing hormone (GnRH) pulse generator occurs to initiate pubertal development. Discussion of the many factors influencing the onset of puberty is beyond the scope of this review and can be found in other publications.[3]

DEFINITIONS

Primary amenorrhea is defined as the lack of menses by the age of 14 years in the absence of secondary sexual characteristics or lack of menses by 15 years in the presence of breast development. From the third-year postmenarche until menopause, menses should occur every 21 to 35 days. Secondary amenorrhea is characterized by the absence of menses for at least 6 months in a postmenarcheal girl. Premature ovarian insufficiency (POI), also known as primary ovarian insufficiency, is defined as lack of menses for at least 4 months associated with elevated serum follicle stimulating hormone (FSH) and low estradiol concentrations obtained twice at least 1 month apart before the age of 40 years.[4,5]

Conditions associated with primary amenorrhea include (1) hypogonadotropic hypogonadism characterized by low luteinizing hormone (LH) and FSH secretion, (2) hypergonadotropic hypogonadism (HH) associated with increased LH and FSH secretion and gonadal dysfunction, (3) anatomic variants of Müllerian duct derivatives, and (4) transient/functional hypogonadism.[3] This review will focus on ovarian and anatomic causes for primary amenorrhea.

BACKGROUND

HH typically reflects gonadal dysfunction. One cause of HH is POI. POI is associated with ovarian dysgenesis, accelerated depletion of primordial follicles, or ovarian dysfunction. This heterogeneous condition exists in nonsyndromic and syndromic forms. Aberrant gonadal differentiation associated with 46,XY or 46,XX differences in sex development (DSD), sex chromosome abnormalities, or defects in gonadal steroidogenesis may present with delayed puberty and/or primary amenorrhea.[6]

In female individuals, the X chromosome plays a pivotal role in normal gonadal development, ovarian folliculogenesis, oocyte maturation, hormone regulation, and sex-specific gene expression profiles. Numerical and structural X chromosome abnormalities or pathogenic changes in genes essential for gonadal development, gonadal steroidogenesis, follicular development, and ovulation are associated with POI.[7,8] In somatic cells, most X-linked genes are expressed from a single active X chromosome. However, the presence of 2 structurally and functionally active X chromosomes is essential for oogenesis.

TURNER SYNDROME AND X CHROMOSOME MONOSOMY

Monosomy X (45,X), also known as Turner syndrome (TS), is the most common cause of primary amenorrhea. TS affects approximately 1 in 2500 live-born girls and is characterized by accelerated follicular atresia during fetal development, often resulting in streak gonads at birth.[9] Other clinical manifestations include characteristic physical appearance, lymphedema in infancy, short stature, congenital heart defects, hearing loss, and skeletal and kidney anomalies. Affected individuals have infantile internal and external genitalia and generally fail to undergo spontaneous puberty.[10] Approximately 50% of patients with TS have a 45,X chromosome complement in most cells through their body, whereas the remaining 50% have mosaicism for a cell line with either a normal 46,XX or 46,XY chromosome complement, trisomy X (47,XXX), or one normal X and a structurally abnormal X chromosome in their cells. Mosaicism for multiple abnormal cell lines is also common. TS phenotype is more commonly observed in patients with abnormalities affecting the short (*P*) arm of an X chromosome. Haploinsufficiency for X-linked genes such as *BMP15*, critical for ovarian development and maintenance of germ cells, is likely responsible for gonadal dysgenesis in individuals with 45,X and structural Xp aberrations. Clinical manifestations of mosaic 45,X are extremely variable, ranging from unaffected individuals to infertility or secondary amenorrhea, or to a more severe presentation such as primary amenorrhea and characteristic clinical stigmata of TS.[10]

Rearrangements involving the Xq13, Xq21, and Xq23-Xq27 bands are also associated with Turner or Turner-like phenotype. Multiple molecular studies showed that most of these rearrangements do not involve gene-coding sequences, thus broken structural chromosome integrity is thought to be responsible for the pathogenesis of POI in such cases.[7]

DIFFERENCES IN SEX DEVELOPMENT

Conditions affecting gonadal differentiation or steroidogenesis (**Table 1**) are also associated with delayed puberty or primary amenorrhea.[6] At birth, individuals with 46,XY complete gonadal dysgenesis (Swyer syndrome), 46,XY complete androgen insensitivity (CAIS) associated with androgen receptor (*AR*) variants, and 46,XY Leydig cell hypoplasia (*LHCGR*) may be categorized as girls. CAIS is characterized by breast development and primary amenorrhea due to aromatization of testosterone to estrogens. Individuals with gonadal dysgenesis and *LHCGR* may present with delayed puberty.

Table 1
Genes associated with delayed puberty, primary amenorrhea, or premature ovarian insufficiency

XY and XX Gonadal Differentiation	XY-DSD	XX^a-Ovarian Development	XX-Chromosome Pairing and Synapsis	XX-DNA Damage Repair	XX-Defects in Ovarian Steroidogenesis
DHH	*AKRC2, AKRC4*	*BMPR2*	*RAD51 B*	*BRCA2*	*BMP15*
DMRT1	*AR*	*FIGLA*	*STAG3*	*HFM1*	*CYP11A1*
DMRT2	*HSD17B3*	*GATA4*	*SYCE1*	*MCM8*	*CYP17A1*
FOXL2	*SOX9*	*LHX8*	*SYCP1*	*MCM9*	*CYP19A1*
NR2F2	*SRD5A2*	*NOBOX*	*SYCP2*	*MEIOB*	*FSHR*
NR5A1	*SRY*	*NOTCH2*	*SYCP3*	*MSH4*	*LGCGR*
RSPO1		*NUP107*		*MSH5*	*POR*
SOX9		*SOHLH1*		*TP63*	*STAR*
SRY		*SOHLH2*		*WDR62*	
WNT4		*WT1*		*XRCC4*	
WT1				*ZSWIM7*	
ZNRF3					

^a In the presence of 2 X chromosomes, the expression of multiple transcriptional regulators triggers ovarian development. Heterozygous and homozygous variants in these genes have been identified in patients with ovarian dysgenesis.

Individuals with 46,XY and 17β-hydroxysteroid dehydrogenase type 3 (*HSD17B3*) deficiency, 5-α-reductase type 2 (*SRD5A2*) deficiency, or steroidogenic factor-1 (*NR5A1*) variants may be viewed as girls at birth; however, these individuals virilize at puberty due to increased testosterone production.[11] Individuals with variants in the P450-oxidoreductase (*POR*), steroidogenic acute regulatory protein (*STAR*), cholesterol desmolase (*CYP11A1*), or 17α-hydroxylase/17,20-lyase (*CYP17A1*) genes may present with female external genitalia and delayed puberty regardless of sex chromosome karyotype due to the inability to synthesize any sex steroids, testosterone, or estradiol.

MÜLLERIAN AGENESIS

Individuals with agenesis of the Müllerian structures, known as Mayer-Rokitansky-Küster-Hauser (MRKH) syndrome, typically present with normal breast development and primary amenorrhea. Clinically, type 1 is characterized by agenesis of the uterus, fallopian tubes, cervix, and upper vagina, and type 2 is associated with renal, skeletal, auditory, and/or cardiac valve abnormalities in addition to aberrant Müllerian duct structures. Deleterious variants have been identified in *WNT4* and *HNF1B* genes in a small cohort of patients with MRKH.[12]

OTHER CAUSES OF PREMATURE OVARIAN INSUFFICIENCY

Ovarian and oocyte development is coordinated by a significant number of autosomal genes responsible for ovarian differentiation, neuroendocrine signaling, adrenal and gonadal steroidogenesis, recruitment and activation of primordial follicles, repair of DNA damage, and maintenance of genomic integrity during mitosis and meiosis of germ cells.[8,13,14] Through genome-wide analyses of single-nucleotide variants (SNVs) and identification of copy number alterations in large cohorts of affected individuals, novel genes involved in the etiology of gonadal dysgenesis have been discovered (see **Table 1**).

During meiosis, numerous programmed DNA double-strand breaks and the subsequent recombination facilitate synapsis and segregation of homologous chromosomes in germ cells. Pathogenic variants in several genes, known to play a role in chromosome pairing and synapsis and response to DNA damage, have been found in patients with POI (see **Table 1**). Meiotic checkpoint mechanisms safeguard DNA integrity to ensure the production of gametes with the correct chromosome complement, whereas the inability to repair DNA breaks activates apoptosis to eliminate damaged germ cells.

Pathogenic SNVs in several genes associated with syndromic conditions may result in ovarian dysgenesis and POI associated with additional clinical manifestations (**Table 2**). Representative examples include blepharophimosis with ptosis and epicanthus inversus caused by defects in the *FOXL2* gene, Perrault syndrome due to pathogenic variants in the *HSD17B4*, *HARS2*, *CLPP*, *LARS2*, and *C10ORF2* genes, and carbohydrate-deficient glycoprotein syndromes with pathogenic variants in *PMM2*.

Galactosemia is an autosomal recessive disorder of galactose metabolism, caused by pathogenic variants in the *GALK1*, *GALT*, *GALM*, or *GALE* genes. Complications of galactosemia include failure to thrive, jaundice, liver failure in infancy, developmental delay, neuromotor abnormalities, cataracts, and HH. Affected female individuals have numerous oocytes and normal-appearing ovaries at birth with a rapid loss of follicles during puberty followed by early onset amenorrhea.[15]

Another condition associated with POI is CGG trinucleotide repeat expansion in the fragile X messenger ribonucleoprotein (*FMR1*) gene. Approximately 1 per 150 to 300

Table 2
Syndromes associated with delayed puberty, primary amenorrhea, or premature ovarian insufficiency

Syndrome	Chromosomal Anomaly/Genetic Variant	Inheritance Pattern
TS and variants	Monosomy X, structural or numerical variant of X chromosome	Sporadic
Mixed gonadal dysgenesis	45,X/46,XY and variants	Sporadic
Ataxia telangiectasia	ATM	AR
Autoimmune polyendocrinopathy syndrome, type 1	AIRE	AR
Blepharophimosis, ptosis, epicanthus inversus syndrome	FOXL2	AD
Fanconi anemia	FANCA, FANCM, FANCL, FANCD1/BRCA2, and FANCU/XRCC2	AR
Galactosemia	GALT, GALK1, GALM, or GALE	AR
Ovarioleukodystrophy	EIF2B2 and EIF2B4	AR
Perrault syndrome	HSD17B4m HARS2, LARS2, CLPP, C10orf2, CLDN14+SGO2, KIAA039, and ERAL1	AR
Premature aging syndromes	WRN and ANTXR1	AR
Progressive external ophthalmoplegia	POLG	AR
Pseudohypoparathyroidism type 1a	PHP1a	AD
Woodhouse-Sakati syndrome	DCAF17	AR

female individuals has 55 to 200 CGG repeats (premutation alleles) at the 5'-untranslated region. Nearly 20% of women heterozygous for a premutation allele have HH with elevated FSH levels and decreased inhibin A, inhibin B, progesterone, and anti-Müllerian hormone (AMH) levels associated with the depletion of ovarian follicles culminating in POI. Affected women are at risk of having a child affected with fragile X syndrome.

Complex interactions between the oocyte, granulosa, and theca cells are essential to generate developmentally competent oocytes. Theca and granulosa cells play a critical role in ovarian steroidogenesis by coordinating endocrine and paracrine signaling, regulating follicle maturation, and ovulation. Androgens synthesized in theca cells undergo aromatization in granulosa cells to produce estrogens. Depletion and/or dysfunction of granulosa cells directly affect the quantity and quality of follicles, leading to POI. Several oocyte-expressed proteins, including GDF9, BMP6, BMP15, and FGF8B, are known to stimulate granulosa cell proliferation and activity. Accumulating evidence suggests that long non-coding RNAs and microRNAs regulate transcription, chromatin status, and mRNA degradation of ovary-expressed genes, and thus coordinate intrafollicle signaling. Altered levels of non-coding RNA in ovaries and plasma appear to correlate with granulosa cell aging and, in the future, could potentially be useful diagnostic and prognostic biomarkers of POI and ovarian longevity.[16,17]

POI can also be due to autoimmune mechanisms. No direct test is reliable for anti-ovarian antibodies. Rather the diagnosis depends on circumstantial evidence of other autoimmune disorders and autoantibodies. Concurrent endocrine autoimmune disorders may affect the thyroid, adrenal, and parathyroid. Associated nonendocrine features include chronic candidiasis, vitiligo, pernicious anemia, and chronic active hepatitis.[18] Autoimmune-related POI can occur as a manifestation of autoimmune polyglandular syndrome. Gonadotoxic cancer treatment, including both chemotherapy and radiation therapy, can cause POI in cancer survivors. In rare instances, primary ovarian tumors and treatment can cause POI.[19]

CLINICAL EVALUATION

Delayed puberty and primary amenorrhea can be due to hypothalamic, pituitary, or gonadal dysfunction. Specific causes include genetic variants, chromosomal anomalies, enzyme defects, hormonal imbalances, tumors, and structural abnormalities. Evaluation of amenorrhea starts with a thorough past medical history, family history, and physical examination (**Fig. 1**). The initial consultation should be conducted with sensitivity, dignity, and respect. This consultation will hopefully initiate an enduring relationship between the young woman and the health-care team. A diagnostic odyssey delaying the diagnosis and frustrating the patient and her family should be avoided. The young woman and her family need to understand the rationale for the questions, the detailed physical examination, and the laboratory studies. Particularly relevant findings include height potential in relation to midparental height, the extent of pubertal development (breast and pubic hair), any signs of androgen excess, and blood pressure.

Based on these initial findings, directed bloodwork and imaging studies can be obtained. Pregnancy tests should be performed in all patients with primary (or secondary) amenorrhea with secondary sexual characteristics to exclude pregnancy. Initial bloodwork includes thyroid function studies, prolactin, FSH, LH, and estradiol

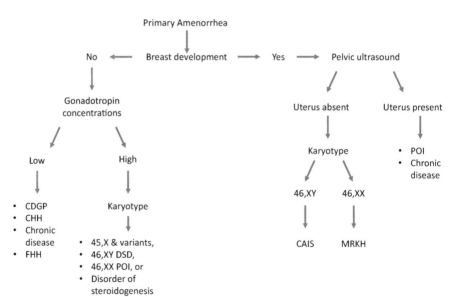

Fig. 1. Flowchart for evaluation of primary amenorrhea. CAIS, complete androgen insensitivity syndrome; CDGP, constitutional delay of growth and puberty; CHH, congenital hypothalamic hypogonadism; DSD, differences in sex development; FHH, functional hypothalamic hypogonadism; MRKH, Mayer-Rokitansky-Küster-Hauser syndrome; POI, premature ovarian insufficiency.

concentrations. If hirsutism, severe cystic acne, or other signs of hyperandrogenism are present, testosterone, 17-hydroxyprogesterone, androstenedione, and dehydro-epiandrosterone sulfate concentrations should be obtained. AMH concentrations provide information regarding ovarian follicular reserve because AMH serves as a gatekeeper for FSH-induced follicular maturation. Low AMH concentrations suggest limited ovarian reserve for girls with TS and for some with idiopathic POI.[20] However, normative ranges are not well established, and variability in AMH concentrations occurs. Hence, AMH determinations have limited usefulness in the diagnosis of POI.

A pelvic ultrasound may be helpful in girls with primary amenorrhea to delineate urogenital anatomy. In some instances, MR imaging or CT imaging will be needed to define specific details of urogenital, renal, and adrenal anatomy. With the exception of cancer survivors, karyotype should be obtained in all individuals.[5] Importantly, karyotype based on 20 white blood cells may not necessarily detect or precisely represent the extent of mosaicism. When clinical findings suggest the diagnosis of TS or a DSD, analysis of 300 interphase cells for the X and Y chromosome by fluorescence in situ hybridization (FISH) is appropriate. In some instances, testing of different tissues from a patient is essential due to varying degrees of mosaicism.

Gonadotropin concentrations and karyotype should be obtained in girls with short stature and subnormal linear growth velocity to assess for TS. With a diagnosis of TS, evaluation for associated comorbidities is recommended, including thyroid function studies, cardiac evaluation, renal ultrasound to assess for horseshoe kidneys, and formal hearing test.[10]

Potential diagnoses for girls with breast development and primary amenorrhea include CAIS and Müllerian duct anomalies. Girls with CAIS have 46,XY karyotype, elevated testosterone concentrations, and absence of Müllerian structures on ultrasound. In patients with CAIS, testes develop but the loss-of-function *AR* variants interfere with androgen signaling leading to undervirilization of the external genitalia. The testes in these individuals secrete AMH leading to regression of Müllerian duct structures. Girls with Müllerian duct anomalies have 46,XX karyotype, normal gonadotropin concentrations, and absence of Müllerian structures on ultrasound; ovarian differentiation and development are typically normal. Additional evaluation is important for girls with Müllerian duct structure due to risk for renal, skeletal, and cardiac anomalies. Müllerian duct aplasia–renal agenesis–cervicothoracic somite dysplasia association consists of uterine hypoplasia or aplasia, short stature, renal abnormalities, and vertebral anomalies.

TREATMENT

Treatment should be guided by the underlying cause of primary amenorrhea. First steps include thorough frank discussions with the individual and her family regarding her specific diagnosis. Learning about subfertility/infertility and associated comorbidities often precipitates sadness, shock, anxiety, poor self-esteem, depression, and adverse effects on sexuality. Open dialog and shared decision-making among the individual, parents, and the health-care team are vital.

Pubertal Induction and Estrogen/Progestogen Therapy

Timely induction of pubertal development is essential. One important goal of estrogen therapy is to mirror typical pubertal progression with breast development and uterine growth. Transdermal estradiol is preferred for the replacement therapy because this approach avoids the first pass through the liver with ensuing deleterious effects on clotting factors. Specifically, estrogens increase production of procoagulant proteins including factor VII, factor VIII, factor X, von Willebrand factor, and fibrinogen. Personal and family histories for increased risk for venous thromboembolic events (VTEs) should be obtained by inquiring about inherited thrombophilias such a Factor V Leiden or prothrombin 2 variants. Deficiencies in protein S, protein C, and antithrombin are also associated with an increased risk for clotting. A thorough medical history is the best approach to assess the risk for inherited thrombophilias. Transdermal estradiol should be used for pubertal induction and maintenance hormone replacement for those with thrombophilias to decrease risks for VTEs.

Initial pubertal induction involves low transdermal estradiol dosage. Transdermal estradiol doses of 3 to 7 mcg/d are achieved by cutting matrix patches (0.014–0.025 mg/24 h) into quarters or eighths. The dose can be increased approximately every 6 months until adult replacement dosage is achieved in 2 to 3 years. The dose can titrated every 6 months to achieve a final dose of 75-100 µg. The starting and final dose varies depending on the degree of estrogen deficiency or development at initiation and by the response to estrogen (guided by the history and physical examination. High-estrogen dosages should be avoided during growth to prevent premature epiphyseal closure in girls who have not yet achieved final adult height and to avoid poor breast development exemplified by prominent nipples with little supporting breast tissue.

For those with severe skin irritation or aversion to the patch, oral estradiol can be used. Oral micronized 17β-estradiol is recommended, prescribed as either weight based (5 mcg/kg/d for the first year and 7.5 mcg/kg/d for the second year) or fixed doses (0.20 mg/d in the first year followed by 0.4–0.5 mg/d in the second year) can be used.[21] Preparations containing conjugated equine estrogens are no longer recommended for pubertal induction or maintenance therapy. Most oral contraceptives contain ethinyl estradiol at higher doses than appropriate for induction of puberty and hence, are not recommended for pubertal induction.[22] Ethinyl estradiol is a synthetic form of 17β-estradiol. Ethinyl estradiol is a "forever" chemical due to its resistance to metabolism; it is not inactivated by 17β-HSD and is not metabolized to estradiol.

After approximately 18 to 24 months of unopposed estrogen therapy, addition of progestogens can be considered. For those with a uterus, progestogens should be initiated to reduce the risk for future endometrial hyperplasia.[5] Progestogens can be introduced earlier if breakthrough vaginal bleeding occurs. Some advocate obtaining pelvic ultrasound studies and initiating progestogen therapy when the uterus appears mature and shows thickening of the endometrial lining.[21] Progestogens are generally unnecessary in those lacking a uterus. Progestins vary in potency and can be administered by transdermal, oral, or uterine routes. Although increased potency may have beneficial effects on withdrawal bleeding, greater progestogenic side effects may develop.

The scarcity of definitive evidence-based data has prompted the use of different regimens for cyclic hormone replacement therapy. Sequential oral or transdermal estrogen/progestin administration ensures monthly vaginal withdrawal bleeding. One regimen for cyclic vaginal withdrawal bleeding consists of transdermal estradiol patch application (0.05–0.1 mg) or 2 mg of oral 17β-estradiol, alone for approximately 2 weeks. During the third week, in addition to estradiol, either oral medroxyprogesterone acetate (10 mg) or oral micronized progesterone (100–200 mg) can be added for 7 to 10 days each month. Cessation of both estrogen and progestin for 4 to 7 days is typically followed by a withdrawal bleed. This schedule can be repeated monthly to ensure monthly menses and reduce the risk for endometrial hyperplasia.

Another regimen involves continuous 100 mcg transdermal estradiol and treatment with 10 mg oral medroxyprogesterone or oral micronized progesterone (100–200 mg) daily for 12 days each month; this regimen was associated with improved bone mineral density in a small double-blind, single-center, placebo-controlled clinical trial.[23] Oral contraceptive pills are often used for convenience but should only be used after an adolescent has completed pubertal development because the estradiol dose is excessive for pubertal initiation. Contraception should be utilized by those at risk of undesired pregnancies because some patients may have sporadic ovulation.[24,25]

Breakthrough bleeding may occur more commonly with the continuous regimen. For some, continuous transdermal estradiol in conjunction with a levonorgestrel intrauterine device may be optimal.

Adolescents with defects in steroidogenesis or XY DSD generally require estrogen treatment. Individuals with *POR*, *STAR*, *CYP11A1*, and *CYP17A1* variants and those with gonadal dysgenesis cannot synthesize sex steroids. Hence, estradiol treatment is needed for pubertal induction. Progestogen treatment needs to be added if a uterus is present. Individuals with disorders affecting steroidogenesis need to undergo further evaluation to determine if glucocorticoid and mineralocorticoid treatment is necessary. Due to the high risk for gonadal malignancy, gonadectomy is appropriate for individuals with 46,XY gonadal dysgenesis or mosaic TS with a Y chromosome.

If a Y chromosome is present, gonadectomy is necessary because of the increased risk for in situ neoplastic changes, gonadoblastoma, or dysgerminoma. For patients with 46,XY DSD, the appropriate timing for gonadectomy should be individualized. For patients with CAIS, the lower risk for gonadal malignancy allows leaving gonads in situ to permit spontaneous pubertal breast development. Following breast development, individuals with CAIS need to consider the increased risk for gonadal neoplasia and contemplate undergoing gonadectomy.[26]

Following gonadectomy, maintenance estrogen therapy is needed. In some instances, vaginoplasty and/or vaginal dilatation are helpful to enable sexual function. Compassionate discussions about infertility, sexuality, and abnormal sex chromosomes should be unhurried with sensitivity to the individual's specific needs, concerns, and questions. Health-care providers can review these topics at subsequent visits to address additional concerns and questions. Additional counseling support may be beneficial.

For those 46,XY individuals with *17HSDB3*, *SRD5A2*, or *NR5A1* variants who have been raised as girls, comprehensive multifaceted discussions are warranted. These individuals are considered to be girls at birth; they may virilize with the development of clitoromegaly at the onset of puberty. In the past, such individuals typically continued with female gender and sex; gonadectomy and estrogen hormone replacement encompassed the usual treatment regimen. When these individuals present as virilized girls with primary amenorrhea, discussion regarding gender identity is important and relevant.[27] With increased recognition of these steroidogenic disorders affecting testosterone synthesis, affected patients are being identified in the neonatal period and raised as boys.

Adolescents with congenital absence of the uterus who have normal ovarian function do not require hormonal replacement therapy.[28] As noted above, additional testing is necessary to identify associated anomalies. Uterine transplants are a potential option for these women. Adoption and use of surrogates are alternatives for creating a family. Self vaginal dilatation and/or surgical interventions such as vaginoplasty may be needed for normal sexual function.

BONE HEALTH

Estrogen deficiency is associated with impaired bone mineral density (BMD) and increased risk of fractures attributed to osteoclast activation, decreased intestinal calcium absorption, and increased urinary calcium excretion. Indeed, girls with TS have an increased fracture risk compared to healthy individuals. Monitoring of BMD using dual X-ray absorptiometry (DEXA) scans should be initiated during adolescence. In addition to estrogen treatment, other factors contributing to bone health such as optimal vitamin D and calcium intake as well as regular weight-bearing exercise should be discussed and encouraged.

GONAD STATUS, FERTILITY POTENTIAL, AND FERTILITY PRESERVATION

Fertility options remain limited for women with HH. Talking about adoption as an option is appropriate. Oocyte preservation is possible in some girls with TS especially those who have experienced spontaneous pubertal development or have mosaic karyotypes. Ovarian cryopreservation is increasingly available for girls with cancer undergoing treatment with gonadotoxic agents. Individuals with complete gonadal dysgenesis are typically infertile. Those with an intact uterus may be able to bear children after donor oocyte implantation and hormonal support.

BEHAVIORAL HEALTH AND SEXUALITY

Learning that subfertility/infertility will likely occur can be devastating for the individual and family. Concerns regarding medical interventions, potential side effects, social isolation, and new hurdles for future expectations arise. Individuals and families worry about being different. They agonize that sharing this information will only bring embarrassment, shaming, and humiliation. Ongoing candid conversations between the individual (with or without parents) and the health-care team to discuss sexuality in the context of the specific medical condition are essential. Dialog and education regarding body perceptions and sexuality can only improve personal satisfaction and contentment in adulthood. Most youth with DSD self-identify along the binary but some explore variations in gender identity.

TRANSITION TO ADULT HEALTH CARE

Planning for transition from pediatric to adult care providers begins several years before the transition actually occurs. Adolescents need know about their diagnosis, treatment details, and family planning options. The pediatric/adolescent health-care provider should encourage straightforward conversations about hormone replacement therapy, bone health, romantic relationships, and family planning. Transition is a proactive and interactive process culminating in the transfer of care to knowledgeable adult health-care providers.

SUMMARY

Numerous causes are associated with primary amenorrhea and POI. Herein, we have primarily focused on HH including X chromosome anomalies, monogenic disorders, autoimmune conditions, and steroidogenic defects. Regardless of the cause, prompt recognition to avoid delayed diagnosis coupled with timely sensitive evaluation and communication is essential. Future research is crucial to augment the limited evidence-based data currently available to enable optimal personalized hormone replacement therapy. Comprehensive communication between the pediatric and adult providers will facilitate transition of health care as the young adult assumes responsibility for her own care.

CLINICS CARE POINTS

- Definitions
  - Primary amenorrhea is the lack of menses by the age of 14 years in the absence of secondary sexual characteristics or lack of menses by the age of 15 years in the presence of breast development.
  - POI is lacking menses for at least 4 months associated with elevated serum FSH and low estradiol concentrations obtained twice at least 1 month apart before the age of 40 years.
- The initial consultation should be conducted with sensitivity, dignity, and respect. This consultation will hopefully initiate an enduring relationship between the young woman and the health-care team.
- A diagnostic odyssey delaying the diagnosis and frustrating the patient and her family should be avoided.
- Shared decision-making regarding the initiation of estradiol hormone replacement therapy is essential and greatly benefits the patient.
- Perform assessments for additional clinical features as appropriate, for example cardiac echocardiology and renal ultrasound in girls diagnosed with TS.
- Engage in sensitive discussions regarding sexuality, potential for fertility, fertility preservation, and ways to have a family.
- Consider bone health.
- Prepare individual for transition to adult care

DISCLOSURE

The authors have no conflicts of interest to report.

REFERENCES

1. Cabrera SM, Bright GM, Frane JW, et al. Age of thelarche and menarche in contemporary US females: a cross-sectional analysis. J Pediatr Endocrinol Metab 2014;27:47–51.
2. Ljubicic ML, Busch AS, Upners EN, et al. A biphasic pattern of reproductive hormones in healthy female infants: the COPENHAGEN Minipuberty Study. J Clin Endocrinol Metab 2022;107:2598–605.
3. Argente J, Dunkel L, Kaiser UB, et al. Molecular basis of normal and pathological puberty: from basic mechanisms to clinical implications. Lancet Diabetes Endocrinol 2023;11:203–16.
4. Pitts S, DiVasta AD, Gordon CM. Evaluation and management of amenorrhea. JAMA 2021;326(19):1962–3.
5. European Society for Human Reproduction and Embryology (ESHRE) Guideline Group on POI, Webber L, Davies M, Anderson R, et al. ESHRE Guideline: management of women with premature ovarian insufficiency. Hum Reprod 2016;31: 926–37.
6. Ahmed SF, Achermann J, Alderson J, et al. Society for endocrinology UK Guidance on the initial evaluation of a suspected difference or disorder of sex development (Revised 2021). Clin Endocrinol 2021;95:818–40.
7. Yatsenko SA, Wood-Trageser M, Chu T, et al. A high-resolution X chromosome copy-number variation map in fertile females and women with primary ovarian insufficiency. Genet Med 2019;21(10):2275–84.

8. Yatsenko SA, Rajkovic A. Genetics of human female infertility. Biol Reprod 2019; 101:549–66.
9. Nielsen J, Wohlert M. Chromosome abnormalities found among 34,910 newborn children: results from a 13-year incidence study in Arhus, Denmark. Hum Genet 1991;87:81–3.
10. Gravholt CH, Viuff M, Just J, et al. The Changing Face of Turner Syndrome. Endocr Rev 2023;44:33–69.
11. Bergougnoux A, Gaspari L, Soleirol M, et al. In adolescent girls, virilization at puberty may reveal a 46,XY disorder of sexual development. Endocr Connect 2023; 12(12):e230267.
12. Mikhael S, Dugar S, Morton M, et al. Genetics of agenesis/hypoplasia of the uterus and vagina: narrowing down the number of candidate genes for Mayer-Rokitansky-Küster-Hauser Syndrome. Hum Genet 2021;140:667–80.
13. Ke H, Tang S, Guo T, et al. Landscape of pathogenic mutations in premature ovarian insufficiency. Nat Med 2023;29(2):483–92.
14. Ding X, Gong X, Fan Y, et al. DNA double-strand break genetic variants in patients with premature ovarian insufficiency. J Ovarian Res 2023;16(1):135.
15. Thakur M, Feldman G, Puscheck EE. Primary ovarian insufficiency in classic galactosemia: current understanding and future research opportunities. J Assist Reprod Genet 2018;35(1):3–16.
16. Nouri N, Shareghi-Oskoue O, Aghebati-Maleki L, et al. Role of miRNAs interference on ovarian functions and premature ovarian failure. Cell Commun Signal 2022;20(1):198.
17. Zhang JH, Chen JH, Guo B, et al. Recent insights into noncoding RNAs in primary ovarian insufficiency: focus on mechanisms and treatments. J Clin Endocrinol Metab 2023;108(8):1898–908.
18. Reato G, Morlin L, Chen S, et al. Premature ovarian failure in patients with autoimmune Addison's disease: clinical, genetic, and immunological evaluation. J Clin Endocrinol Metab 2011;96:E1255–61.
19. Foster KL, Lee DJ, Witchel SF, Gordon CM. Ovarian Insufficiency and Fertility Preservation During and After Childhood Cancer Treatment. J Adolesc Young Adult Oncol 2024. https://doi.org/10.1089/jayao.2023.0111.
20. Hagen CP, Fischer MB, Mola G, et al. AMH and other markers of ovarian function in patients with Turner syndrome - a single center experience of transition from pediatric to gynecological follow up. Front Endocrinol 2023;14: 1173600.
21. Donaldson M, Kriström B, Ankarberg-Lindgren C, et al. Optimal pubertal induction in girls with turner syndrome using either oral or transdermal estradiol: a proposed modern strategy. Horm Res Paediatr 2019;91:153–63.
22. Dowlut-McElroy T, Shankar RK. The care of adolescents and young adults with turner syndrome: a pediatric and adolescent gynecology perspective. J Pediatr Adolesc Gynecol 2022;35:429–34.
23. Popat VB, Calis KA, Kalantaridou SN, et al. Bone mineral density in young women with primary ovarian insufficiency: results of a three-year randomized controlled trial of physiological transdermal estradiol and testosterone replacement. J Clin Endocrinol Metab 2014;99:3418–26.
24. Matthews D, Bath L, Högler W, et al. Hormone supplementation for pubertal induction in girls. Arch Dis Child 2017;102:975–80.
25. Klein KO, Phillips SA. Review of Hormone Replacement Therapy in Girls and Adolescents with Hypogonadism. J Pediatr Adolesc Gynecol 2019;32: 460–8.

26. Patel V, Casey RK, Gomez-Lobo V. Timing of gonadectomy in patients with complete androgen insensitivity syndrome-current recommendations and future directions. J Pediatr Adolesc Gynecol 2016;29:320–5.
27. Bonnet E, Winter M, Mallet D, et al. Changes in the clinical management of 5α-reductase type 2 and 17β-hydroxysteroid dehydrogenase type 3 deficiencies in France. Endocr Connect 2023;12(3):e220227.
28. Fitzgerald S, Gordon CM, Fleischman A. Amenorrhea, the polycystic ovary syndrome and hirsutism. In: Katzman DK, Gordon CM, Callahan ST, et al, editors. *Neinstein's adolescent and young adult health care: a practical guide.* 7th edition. Philadelphia: Wolters Kluwer; 2023. p. 488–500.

Hormone Therapy During Infancy or Early Childhood for Patients with Hypogonadotropic Hypogonadism, Klinefelter or Turner Syndrome: Has the Time Come?

Elodie Fiot, MD[a], Juliane Léger, MD, PhD[a,b],
Laetitia Martinerie, MD, PhD[a,b,c],*

KEYWORDS

- Minipuberty • Androgens • Estrogens • Gonadotropins
- Hypogonadotropic hypogonadism • Klinefelter syndrome • Turner syndrome

KEY POINTS

- Mimicking minipuberty in CHH with gonadotropins.
- Low dose androgens during infancy in Klinefelter syndrome.
- Low dose oestrogens during infancy in Turner syndrome
- Managing patients unable to produce sex steroids using gonadotropins to mimic minipuberty in hypogonadotropic hypogonadism, or sex steroids in patients with Klinefelter or Turner syndrome, is promising.
- There is a need to pursue research in this area, with large prospective cohorts and long-term data before these treatments can be routinely considered.

INTRODUCTION

Understanding the physiologic secretion of gonadotropins and sex steroids throughout development[1,2] has led to a new area of potential therapeutic windows.[3]

[a] Endocrinologie Pédiatrique, Centre de Référence des Maladies Endocriniennes Rares de la Croissance et du Développement, Hôpital Universitaire Robert-Debré, Paris 75019, France; [b] Université Paris Cité, Faculté de Santé, UFR de Médecine, Paris, France; [c] Université Paris-Saclay, Inserm, Physiologie et Physiopathologie Endocriniennes, Le Kremlin-Bicêtre 94276, France
* Corresponding author. Pediatric Endocrinology Department CHU Robert Debré, 48 boulevard Sérurier, 75019 Paris, France.
E-mail address: laetitia.martinerie@aphp.fr

Endocrinol Metab Clin N Am 53 (2024) 307–320
https://doi.org/10.1016/j.ecl.2024.02.003
0889-8529/24/© 2024 Elsevier Inc. All rights reserved.

endo.theclinics.com

During fetal development, activation of gonadal secretion is initially under the control of human chorionic gonadotropin (hCG). During the first trimester, anti-Müllerian hormone (AMH), synthesized by Sertoli cells, and sex steroids, principally testosterone, biosynthesized by Leydig cells, drive the differentiation of internal and external genitalia. The hypothalamic–pituitary secretions of gonadotropin releasing hormone (GnRH), luteinizing hormone (LH), and follicle-stimulating hormone (FSH) start around the 16th week of gestation in humans.[4] From the second trimester and on, gonadal secretions will be controlled by hypothalamic–pituitary stimulation. The gonadotropic axis follows a triphasic pattern of activation (**Fig. 1**, for the gonadotropic axis throughout development in males). The first activation occurs during the fetal period. A second activation phase is observed during the neonatal period, called minipuberty,[1,2] which lasts from 2 postnatal weeks in full-term newborns (delayed in preterm infants) until a few months after birth (for a shorter period in males compared to females). The third phase starts at puberty. Each of these activation phases is important for gonadal development and hormone secretion, development of genital organs and secondary sexual characteristics, as well as to prepare future fertility. Sex steroid secretion during minipuberty and infancy has also been related to neurodevelopment, metabolic, and bone health. Several studies have evaluated the impact of gonadotropins or sex steroid supplementation in different conditions affecting sex steroid production prior to puberty. We will review herein the relevance of gonadotropin treatment in hypogonadotropic hypogonadism in male patients and sex steroid treatment in patients with Klinefelter syndrome (KS) or Turner syndrome (TS) during infancy and early childhood.

Male Patients with Congenital Hypogonadotropic Hypogonadism

Congenital hypogonadotropic hypogonadism (CHH) is a group of rare diseases characterized by inadequate secretion of gonadotropins during physiologic activation periods of the gonadotropic axis. Clinically, CHH in males may be associated with neonatal clinical signs (micropenis, cryptorchidism in boys in about half of the cases).[5] The minipuberty provides a brief window of opportunity to diagnose CHH. Typically, low testosterone, LH, and FSH levels are reported.[5] AMH levels, however, may be

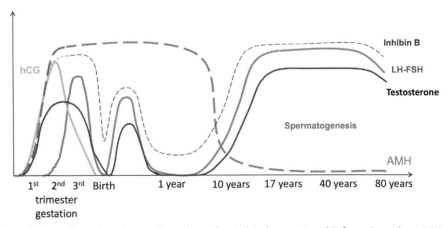

Fig. 1. Gonadotropic axis secretions throughout development and infancy in males. AMH, anti-Müllerian hormone; FSH, follicle-stimulating hormone; hCG, human chorionic gonadotropin; LH, luteinizing hormone.

low or partially maintained.[6] The diagnosis is sometimes only evoked in case of pubertal delay or pubertal maturation arrest in the adolescent.

Different therapeutic options for pubertal induction have been described for CHH patients, but we lack the necessary larger randomized trials to define the best approaches. Since there is no report of decreased follicular reserve[7] and fertility induction and pregnancy rates are high in women with CHH, there is currently no evidence of a beneficial impact of gonadotropins to induce puberty rather than the use of sex steroid in this population.[5,7]

Studies have demonstrated that physiologic gonadal activation by gonadotropins during male puberty is associated with a better outcome for spermatogenesis[8,9] and may offer important psychological reassurance in adolescents and enhance self-confidence.[8]

Pretreatment with FSH alone in case of severe GnRH deficiency has proved to increase inhibin B levels—a marker of Sertoli cell function—and testicular volume, consistent with proliferation of Sertoli cells.[10,11]

Based on these results and the fact that testicular volume and inhibin B levels prior to pubertal induction correlate positively with a better spermatogenic outcome,[12,13] some teams suggested that treatment by gonadotropins during the neonatal period to mimic minipuberty could improve pubertal induction of spermatogenesis and fertility outcome in adulthood.

Treatment with gonadotropins during the neonatal period

To date, hormonal therapy during the neonatal period has only been offered to CHH male patients exhibiting micropenis and/or cryptorchidism. The main goal is to increase penile length and when possible, stimulate testicular volume.

For penile enlargement and enhancement of scrotal development, the usual practice consists of the administration of 2 to 4 doses of intramuscular testosterone enanthate injection, 25 to 50 mg every 2 to 4 weeks.[14] Few case series have been published, as summarized by Mason and colleagues.[14]

However, androgen therapy does not stimulate testicular volume and has no impact on cryptorchidism. During this period in life, serum gonadotropin and testicular hormone levels (testosterone, inhibin B, and AMH) increase, and penile length and testicular volume grow.[15] Testicular volume is a reflection of the increase in the number of immature Sertoli cells[6] in response to FSH. Since these cells only weakly express the androgen receptor in infants, LH-induced endogenous testosterone does not mature the Sertoli cells or activate spermatogenesis.[16] Given that the number of Sertoli cells correlates with sperm-producing capacity later in life, the minipuberty may prepare for future reproductive ability.[11,17] This gives an argument to discuss replacement therapy with gonadotropins in CHH boys.[6]

In addition, hCG therapy alone or in combination with nasal spray of GnRH has been shown to treat cryptorchidism in neonates and prepubertal boys.[18] As cryptorchidism is a factor of poor prognosis for adult fertility and testicular malignancy,[19] gonadotropins may represent an alternative to surgery.

Main and colleagues reported the clinical and biological effects of subcutaneous injections of recombinant luteinizing hormone (rLH) and recombinant follicle stimulating hormone (rFSH) during the first year of life in a CHH boy with micropenis. The treatment led to an increase in penile size from 1.6 to 2.4 cm as well as a 170% increase in testicular volume and inhibin B levels.[20] Bougnères and colleagues reported the use of gonadotropin infusion by pump for 6 months in 2 neonates (1 with isolated CHH and 1 with combined pituitary hormone deficiency). The treatment allowed penile length to increase as well as testicular growth and an increase in testosterone, AMH, and inhibin

Table 1
Studies reporting the use of gonadotropins to mimic minipuberty in congenital hypogonadotropic hypogonadism boys

Reference	n	Age at Treatment Initiation	Treatment	Pump	Clinical Effect	Biological Effect
Main et al,[20] 2002	1	7.9 mo	rhFSH 20 IU sc twice weekly rhLH 21.3 IU sc twice weekly	No	↑ Testicular volume by 170% ↑ Penile length 1.6–2.4 cm	↑ Inhibin B ↑ Estradiol Testosterone undetectable
Bougnères et al,[21] 2008	2	2 and 5 mo	rhFSH 67–125 IU/d rhLH 50–56 IU/d	Yes	↑ Testicular volume 0.5–2.1 mL ↑ Penile length 8–21 mm and 12–48 mm	↑ Inhibin B ↑ AMH ↑ Testosterone
Sarfati et al,[27] 2015	1	1 mo	rhFSH 75 IU/d rhLH 75 IU/d	Yes	↑ Testicular volume 0.33–2.3 mL ↑ Penile length 15–38 mm	
Lambert & Bougnères,[24] 2016	8	0.25–11 mo	rhFSH 75–150 IU/d rhLH 50 IU/d	Yes	↑ Testicular volume to 1.27 mL ↑ Testis descent 70% at the end ↑ Penile length mean + 18.9 mm	↑ Inhibin B ↑ AMH ↑ Testosterone
Stoupa et al,[23] 2017	5	3–5.5 mo	rhFSH 75 IU/d rhLH 75 IU/d	Yes	↑ Penile length from 13.8 ± 4.5–42.6 ± 5 mm	↑ Testosterone to 3.5 ± 4.06 ng/mL ↑ Inhibin B from 94.8 ± 74.9–469.4 ± 282.5 pg/mL ↑ AMH from 49.6 ± 30.6–142 ± 76.5 ng/mL

Study	N	Age	Treatment		Outcomes	Hormone markers
Kohva et al,[26] 2019	5	0.7–4.2 mo	rhFSH 3.4–7.5 UI/kg/week in 2–3 sc Testosterone 25 mg/month 3 mo	No	↑ Penile length mean 17.2–28.8 mm	↑ Inhibin B (transient)
Papadimitriou et al,[25] 2019	10	2.3–9.4 mo	rhFSH 150 UI/d rhLH 75 UI/d	No	↑ Testicular volume to 1.5 mL ↑ Testis descent 100% at the end ↑ Penile length from 2 to 3.8 cm	↑ Inhibin B 27.8–365 ng/mL ↑ AMH 1.54–150 ng/mL ↑ Testosterone 0.02–3.3 ng/mL
Avril et al,[22] 2022	35	5.1 ± 3.5 mo	rhFSH 75 UI/d rhLH 75 UI/d (n = 18)	Yes	↑ Testicular volume ↑ Testis descent ↑ Penile length	↑↑ AMH 463.4 ± 190.6–1375 ± 395.2 pmol/L ↑↑ Inhibin B 68.31 ± 50.90–522.9 ± 204.9 ng/mL ↑ Testosterone 0.05 ± 0.09–3.25 ± 2.28 ng/mL
		13 ± 17.7 mo	rhFSH 25 UI × 3/week rhCG 260 UI × 2/week (n = 17)	No	↑ Testicular volume ↑ Testis descent 50% at the end ↑ Penile length	↑ AMH 246.6 ± 163.6–679.6 ± 330.9 pmol/L ↑ Inhibin B 61.60 ± 54.70–259.7 ± 204.0 ↑↑ Testosterone 0.12 ± 0.07–6.05 ± 4.84 ng/mL

Abbreviation: rhFSH, recombinant human follicle stimulating hormone; rhLH, recombinant human luteinizing hormone.

B levels.[21] Six other clinical case series have since been reported, demonstrating similar results (**Table 1**).[20–27] Recently, Avril and colleagues analyzed retrospectively the clinical and biological efficacy of 2 gonadotropin treatment regimens during minipuberty. The authors compared the administration of gonadotropins during the first months of life using either subcutaneous injections 5 times per week (recombiant human chorionic gonadotropin [rhCG] and rFSH), or subcutaneous continuous infusion by pump (rLH and rFSH).[22] Thirty-five patients were included, which represent the largest cohort to date of CHH boys treated during minipuberty with gonadotropins. In both groups, results showed a significant increase in penile length and width, testosterone, AMH, and inhibin B levels, as well as improved testicular descent. Recombinant hCG injections induced higher testosterone levels than continuous LH infusion but frequently above the upper limit of normal. The low-dose rFSH regimen (equivalent to 10 IU/day) permitted AMH and inhibin B levels to reach the normal range for minipuberty. Finally, no additional benefit was seen with the 6 month regimen compared to the 3 month regimen. Thus, the current best treatment option for gonadotropins would be to use recombinant LH and FSH by pump for a 3-month period. However, this will need to be evaluated prospectively.

In addition, only results on the short term have been published. Although the results from these studies are promising by showing that gonadotropins allow testicular descent, increase testicular volume, and probably stimulate Sertoli cell proliferation, there are currently no long-term follow-up data on these markers, on future pubertal induction, and ability to produce sperm. Thus, these studies should be considered preliminary, and more data are warranted before these treatments can be offered aside from specialized centers and clinical trials.

In the future, discussion might also arise on the purpose of minipuberty in girls, and whether mimicking minipuberty or pubertal induction by gonadotropins could have a rationale.

Klinefelter Syndrome

KS is the most common sex chromosomal aneuploidy, with an estimated prevalence of 1:650 male births. Affected males are characterized by hypergonadotropic hypogonadism and infertility but can also have associated comorbidities including neurocognitive deficits, low bone mass, hypotonia, and an adverse cardiometabolic profile. Androgen therapy is the cornerstone of treatment in adolescents and adults.[28]

Most studies regarding secretion of testosterone in KS boys during minipuberty have found on average lower levels.[29] Clinical characteristics such as micropenis and cryptorchidism are also suggestive of testosterone deficiency in early life.[30] As the development of noninvasive prenatal screening allows earlier diagnosis of boys with KS, there is a great interest to understand whether androgen administration in early life and childhood could result in improvements of the various manifestations of KS.

Neurodevelopment profile

The neurodevelopmental profile of males with KS includes weaknesses in executive functioning, language-based learning disabilities; neuromotor dysfunction, and muscle hypotonia.[31,32] Full-Scale Intelligence Quotient is 10 to 20 points lower in KS boys than controls.[33] MRI of boys with KS shows that they have a thinner frontal cortex (important for executive functioning)[34] and a reduced hippocampus volume (role in spatial memory).[35]

Some studies underline a relationship between testosterone and brain morphology in the hippocampus and temporal and prefrontal cortex.[36,37] Studies in aging men and men with hypogonadotropic hypogonadism showed that low testosterone is associated with a decline in memory and visual performance, and the initiation of sub-stitutive androgen treatment mitigates these problems.[38] It was thus hypothesized that androgen treatment in early life could improve neurodevelopmental issues in boys with KS.

In several retrospective studies, injections of testosterone enanthate in early infancy and childhood (<6 years) were associated with improvement in various cognitive do-mains including auditory comprehension, expressive ability, and verbal intelli-gence,[39–41] as well as in motor skills.[42] In a cross-sectional retrospective analysis of 111 boys with KS, injections of testosterone enanthate administered before 5 years of age, or between 5 and 10 years of age, were associated with better performances in working memory.[43] In a 2 year double-blind clinical trial in which prepubertal pa-tients were randomized to treatment with oxandrolone or to placebo, hippocampal volume was found to be bigger in the oxandrolone group relative to the placebo group, associated with a better performance in spatial memory tasks.[44] However, Ross and colleagues in a randomized, double-blind, placebo-controlled clinical trial of 84 boys with KS aged between 4 and 12 year old, treated with oxandrolone 0.06 mg/kg/d or placebo for 2 years, and evaluated at 12 and 24 months, found no significant differ-ence between the 2 groups concerning cognitive function and language tests, as well as for working memory and attention tests. On the other hand, a significant improvement in anxiety, depression, and social problems scales was seen, without significant differences in hyperactive or aggressive behaviors.[45] Improvement in behavioral functioning was also confirmed in several other studies.[46,47]

Cardiometabolic profile

Men with KS have an unfavorable body composition, with increased adiposity and decreased muscle mass. Up to half of men with KS have metabolic syndrome.[48] Morbidity and mortality related to cardiometabolic diseases are increased.[49] It was recently recognized that even young boys with KS have a high prevalence of metabolic syndrome, as well as increased adiposity.[50] Testosterone deficiency is known to cause increased adiposity and decreased insulin sensitivity, which are improved with androgens.[51] In a cross-sectional study of prepubertal boys with KS, it was found that testicular function is inversely associated with features of metabolic syndrome.[52]

In a randomized clinical trial of 2 years of oral oxandrolone versus placebo in 93 pre-pubertal children with KS, oxandrolone modestly improved body composition, with lowered percentage of body fat and improved triglyceride levels. Oxandrolone treat-ment was relatively well tolerated, although it did result in bone age advancement and lowered high-density lipoprotein (HDL) cholesterol levels.[50] In a prospective, ran-domized trial, 20 infants with KS between 6 and 15 weeks of age received testosterone cypionate 25 mg intramuscularly monthly for 3 doses versus no treatment. The in-crease in percent fat mass Z-scores was greater in the untreated group than in the treated group. On the other hand, fat-free mass, length Z-score, stretched penile length, and growth velocity were greater in the treated group.

Bone health

Between 25% and 43% of adults with KS have low bone mass.[53] An increased risk of vertebral fractures was recently described. A recent meta-analysis of 1141 KS men observed an improvement in bone mass with testosterone replacement.[54] Androgens mediate their effects on the skeleton via aromatization to estradiol, by a direct effect via the androgen receptor, and by increased muscle mass.[55] In vitro, oxandrolone stimulates osteoblast differentiation.[56] As childhood and adolescence are known crit-ical time windows for building optimal peak bone mass, androgen treatment in early childhood could decrease lifelong rates of osteoporosis and fractures. In a random-ized, double-blind, placebo-controlled clinical trial of oxandrolone (0.06 mg/kg daily; $n = 38$) versus placebo ($n = 40$) for 2 years in boys with KS (ages 4–12 years), the bone health index was higher in the oxandrolone group at 2 years.[57] This result is ex-pected to be independent of estrogen action, as oxandrolone is a non-aromatizable testosterone derivative.

Almost all studies described earlier show positive effect of androgen treatment in childhood in boys with KS on neurodevelopmental issues, cardiovascular profile, and bone health. However, many of them are retrospective studies including few numbers of patients. The timing of treatment is different from one study to another and between patients. Results in studies about the neurodevelopmental profile were generally not adjusted for parental ages, education, and occupation, or for timing of diagnosis. Laboratory tests were not performed in most of these studies, making it difficult to evaluate the relationship between androgen levels and symptoms. More-over, no data are available on the long-term effects of androgen treatment in early life and outcomes (fertility, adult height, etc.). One study reported a higher risk of pubarche and puberty at an early age following oxandrolone treatment in prepubertal boys.[58]

Therefore, these studies should be considered preliminary, and these findings need further validation with longer term studies. There is also a need for additional research to decipher underlying mechanisms leading to clinical symptoms in KS patients in or-der to develop targeted treatment.

Turner Syndrome

TS is a condition characterized by complete or partial absence of one X chromosome, affecting approximately 1 in 2000 to 2500 live-born girls. Aside from short stature and gonadal failure, patients may have several congenital or acquired associated condi-tions and a particular neurocognitive profile.

In healthy girls, estradiol is already secreted by ovaries in the prepubertal period.[59] Studies in girls with TS show that there is an impaired secretion of estradiol in infancy and early childhood.[60] It has been suggested that this prolonged estrogen deficiency may have negative effects across many body systems. Several studies have evaluated benefits of low-dose estrogen replacement during early childhood in this population.

Growth

A double-blind, placebo-controlled trial showed a trend toward a synergistic growth benefit from childhood low-dose estrogen (from a starting dose of 25 ng/kilogram/day) treatment combined with GH treatment, with a modest (2.1 cm) enhancement of adult height.[61] Similarly, an increment in adult height of approximately 3 cm was shown with a combination of low doses of oxandrolone and estrogen (40 ng/kg/day) when treatment was started before puberty but after the age of 8 years.[62] This effect seems due to increased local responsiveness of the skeletal growth plate to insulin-like growth factor 1 (IGF1) and/or GH.

Pubertal development

A randomized, double-blind, placebo-controlled clinical trial of growth hormone (GH) and low-dose ethinyl estradiol (EE) initiated during childhood, from 5 years of age, in a large cohort of girls with TS ($n = 149$) showed that girls who received EE therapy had significantly earlier thelarche and a correspondingly slower tempo of puberty (3.3 vs 2.2 years), without advancement in bone maturation.[63] The near normalization of pu-berty tempo may have positive psychosocial effects as there is a reported association between breast development and positive body image/social adjustment in girls with TS.[64]

Lipid profile

Lipid profile was evaluated in 14 TS girls treated with low-dose estrogen replacement (17β-estradiol, 62.5 μg daily) before age 12 years (mean age 10.5 years) followed by a pubertal induction regimen after age 12 years and compared to 14 TS girls treated with conventional estrogen replacement started after age 12 years (mean age 14 years). After 3 years of treatment, a healthier lipid profile was found in girls treated with low-dose estrogen replacement therapy, with lower total and low-density lipoprotein (LDL) cholesterol, compared with girls treated with the conventional estrogen replacement regimen.[65]

Bone mineral density

Hasegawa and colleagues described bone mineral density in a group of 17 TS patients who started their EE therapy with an ultra-low dosage (1–5 ng/kg/day) from 9.8 to 13.7 years. Bone mineral density (BMD) was significantly lower in these patients compared to BMD of TS patients with spontaneous puberty; but there was no significant difference compared to BMD in TS patients who started conjugated estrogens at the age of 12.2 to 18.7 years, with a minimal initial dose of 0.3125 mg/day, once a week.[66] These results may indicate that ultra-low dosage of estrogens in girls with TS should be started earlier in life.

Cognitive profile

The TS phenotype is characterized by a specific neurocognitive profile of impaired visual-spatial and/or visual-perceptual abilities and difficulty with motor function. In a randomized double-blind study, nonverbal processing speed, motor performance, and verbal and nonverbal memory were significantly better in estrogen-treated girls from 5.0 to 12.0 years of age than in placebo recipients of the same age.[67] Whether these findings will influence the psychoeducational outcome or quality of life of women with TS is not yet known.

Thus, the addition of low doses of estrogen in early childhood in patients with TS could potentially be beneficial. However, these studies have several limitations, mostly the fact that they have been evaluated in small groups of participants, that the dosing and administration of childhood estrogens have not been optimized, and that long-term safety has not been assessed. In the TS Clinical Practice Guidelines published in 2016, the authors suggest not routinely adding very low-dose estrogen supplementation in the prepubertal years to further promote growth.[68] Further studies should be performed.

SUMMARY

New insights into the physiology of gonadotropic axis activation, the role of minipuberty, and of sex steroids during infancy have undoubtedly produced new areas of research and proposed new therapeutic options. Many studies have been conducted to date demonstrating promising results, but most still lack the long-term data needed to assess their full effects and safety. In addition, all these treatments remain off-label. Thus, clinical trials with long-term follow-up are warranted.

In the meantime, families must be informed of the possibility of these treatments and if considered, then patients should be directed to specialized tertiary centers where treatments may be proposed as part of approved clinical trials.

CLINICS CARE POINTS

- Mimicking minipuberty in hypogonadotropic hypogonadism using gonadotropins may avoid surgical management of cryptorchidism and improve fertility outcome.
- Treatment with low-dose androgens during infancy in Klinefelter syndrome may improve neurodevelopment and metabolic issues.
- Treatment with low-dose estrogens during infancy in Turner syndrome may improve growth, neurodevelopment, and metabolic issues.
- The long-term effects of these treatments are not yet known.
- These treatments must be further evaluated in large prospective studies before generalized treatment to all patients must be considered.

DISCLOSURE

The authors declare no conflict of interest regarding the content of this article.

REFERENCES

1. Ljubicic ML, Busch AS, Upners EN, et al. A Biphasic Pattern of Reproductive Hormones in Healthy Female Infants: The COPENHAGEN Minipuberty Study. J Clin Endocrinol Metabol 2022;107(9):2598–605.
2. Busch AS, Ljubicic ML, Upners EN, et al. Dynamic Changes of Reproductive Hormones in Male Minipuberty: Temporal Dissociation of Leydig and Sertoli Cell Activity. J Clin Endocrinol Metabol 2022;107(6):1560–8.
3. Rey RA. Recent advancement in the treatment of boys and adolescents with hypogonadism. Therapeutic Advances in Endocrinology 2022;13. 204201882110656.
4. Clements JA, Reyes FI, Winter JS, et al. Studies on human sexual development. III. Fetal pituitary and serum, and amniotic fluid concentrations of LH, CG, and FSH. J Clin Endocrinol Metab 1976;42(1):9–19.
5. Young J, Xu C, Papadakis GE, et al. Clinical Management of Congenital Hypogonadotropic Hypogonadism. Endocr Rev 2019;40(2):669–710.
6. Bouvattier C, Maione L, Bouligand J, et al. Neonatal gonadotropin therapy in male congenital hypogonadotropic hypogonadism. Nat Rev Endocrinol 2011;8(3): 172–82.
7. Bry-Gauillard H, Larrat-Ledoux F, Levaillant JM, et al. Anti-Müllerian Hormone and Ovarian Morphology in Women With Isolated Hypogonadotropic Hypogonadism/ Kallmann Syndrome: Effects of Recombinant Human FSH. J Clin Endocrinol Metab 2017;102(4):1102–11.
8. Rohayem J, Hauffa BP, Zacharin M, et al. "German Adolescent Hypogonadotropic Hypogonadism Study Group." Testicular growth and spermatogenesis: new goals for pubertal hormone replacement in boys with hypogonadotropic hypogonadism? -a multicentre prospective study of hCG/rFSH treatment outcomes during adolescence. Clin Endocrinol 2017;86(1):75–87.
9. Rastrelli G, Corona G, Mannucci E, et al. Factors affecting spermatogenesis upon gonadotropin-replacement therapy: a meta-analytic study. Andrology 2014;2(6): 794–808.

10. Raivio T, Wikström AM, Dunkel L. Treatment of gonadotropin-deficient boys with recombinant human FSH: long-term observation and outcome. Eur J Endocrinol 2007;156(1):105–11.

11. Dwyer AA, Sykiotis GP, Hayes FJ, et al. Trial of recombinant follicle-stimulating hormone pretreatment for GnRH-induced fertility in patients with congenital hypogonadotropic hypogonadism. J Clin Endocrinol Metab 2013;98(11):E1790–5.

12. Liu PY, Baker HWG, Jayadev V, et al. Induction of spermatogenesis and fertility during gonadotropin treatment of gonadotropin-deficient infertile men: predictors of fertility outcome. J Clin Endocrinol Metab 2009;94(3):801–8.

13. Pitteloud N, Hayes FJ, Dwyer A, et al. Predictors of outcome of long-term GnRH therapy in men with idiopathic hypogonadotropic hypogonadism. J Clin Endocrinol Metab 2002;87(9):4128–36.

14. Mason KA, Schoelwer MJ, Rogol AD. Androgens During Infancy, Childhood, and Adolescence: Physiology and Use in Clinical Practice. Endocr Rev 2020;41(3): bnaa003.

15. Kuiri-Hänninen T, Sankilampi U, Dunkel L. Activation of the hypothalamic-pituitary-gonadal axis in infancy: minipuberty. Horm Res Paediatr 2014;82(2): 73–80.

16. Rey RA, Musse M, Venara M, et al. Ontogeny of the androgen receptor expression in the fetal and postnatal testis: its relevance on Sertoli cell maturation and the onset of adult spermatogenesis. Microsc Res Tech 2009;72(11):787–95.

17. Sharpe RM, McKinnell C, Kivlin C, et al. Proliferation and functional maturation of Sertoli cells, and their relevance to disorders of testis function in adulthood. Reproduction 2003;125(6):769–84.

18. Christiansen P, Müller J, Buhl S, et al. Treatment of cryptorchidism with human chorionic gonadotropin or gonadotropin releasing hormone. A double-blind controlled study of 243 boys. Horm Res 1988;30(4–5):187–92.

19. Hutson JM, Balic A, Nation T, et al. Cryptorchidism. Semin Pediatr Surg 2010; 19(3):215–24.

20. Main KM, Schmidt IM, Toppari J, et al. Early postnatal treatment of hypogonadotropic hypogonadism with recombinant human FSH and LH. Eur J Endocrinol 2002;146(1):75–9.

21. Bougnères P, François M, Pantalone L, et al. Effects of an early postnatal treatment of hypogonadotropic hypogonadism with a continuous subcutaneous infusion of recombinant follicle-stimulating hormone and luteinizing hormone. J Clin Endocrinol Metab 2008;93(6):2202–5.

22. Avril T, Hennocq Q, Lambert AS, et al. Gonadotropin administration to mimic minipuberty in hypogonadotropic males: pump or injections? Endocr Connect 2023; 12(4):e220252.

23. Stoupa A, Samara-Boustani D, Flechtner I, et al. Efficacy and Safety of Continuous Subcutaneous Infusion of Recombinant Human Gonadotropins for Congenital Micropenis during Early Infancy. Horm Res Paediatr 2017;87(2):103–10.

24. Lambert AS, Bougneres P. Growth and descent of the testes in infants with hypogonadotropic hypogonadism receiving subcutaneous gonadotropin infusion. Int J Pediatr Endocrinol 2016;2016:13.

25. Papadimitriou DT, Chrysis D, Nyktari G, et al. Replacement of Male Mini-Puberty. J Endocr Soc 2019;3(7):1275–82.

26. Kohva E, Huopio H, Hietamäki J, et al. Treatment of gonadotropin deficiency during the first year of life: long-term observation and outcome in five boys. Hum Reprod 2019;34(5):863–71.

27. Sarfati J, Bouvattier C, Bry-Gauillard H, et al. Kallmann syndrome with FGFR1 and KAL1 mutations detected during fetal life. Orphanet J Rare Dis 2015;10:71.
28. Gravholt CH, Chang S, Wallentin M, et al. Klinefelter Syndrome: Integrating Genetics, Neuropsychology, and Endocrinology. Endocr Rev 2018;39(4):389–423.
29. Lahlou N, Fennoy I, Ross JL, et al. Clinical and hormonal status of infants with nonmosaic XXY karyotype. Acta Paediatr 2011;100(6):824–9.
30. Ross JL, Samango-Sprouse C, Lahlou N, et al. Early androgen deficiency in infants and young boys with 47,XXY Klinefelter syndrome. Horm Res 2005;64(1): 39–45.
31. Fales CL, Knowlton BJ, Holyoak KJ, et al. Working memory and relational reasoning in Klinefelter syndrome. J Int Neuropsychol Soc 2003;9(6):839–46.
32. Ross JL, Roeltgen DP, Stefanatos G, et al. Cognitive and motor development during childhood in boys with Klinefelter syndrome. Am J Med Genet 2008;146A(6): 708–19.
33. Graham JM, Bashir AS, Stark RE, et al. Oral and written language abilities of XXY boys: implications for anticipatory guidance. Pediatrics 1988;81(6):795–806.
34. Giedd JN, Clasen LS, Wallace GL, et al. XXY (Klinefelter syndrome): a pediatric quantitative brain magnetic resonance imaging case-control study. Pediatrics 2007;119(1):e232–40.
35. Lentini E, Kasahara M, Arver S, et al. Sex differences in the human brain and the impact of sex chromosomes and sex hormones. Cereb Cortex 2013;23(10): 2322–36.
36. Hajszan T, MacLusky NJ, Leranth C. Role of androgens and the androgen receptor in remodeling of spine synapses in limbic brain areas. Horm Behav 2008; 53(5):638–46.
37. Leranth C, Petnehazy O, MacLusky NJ. Gonadal hormones affect spine synaptic density in the CA1 hippocampal subfield of male rats. J Neurosci 2003;23(5): 1588–92.
38. Moffat SD, Zonderman AB, Metter EJ, et al. Longitudinal assessment of serum free testosterone concentration predicts memory performance and cognitive status in elderly men. J Clin Endocrinol Metab 2002;87(11):5001–7.
39. Samango-Sprouse CA, Yu C, Porter GF, et al. A review of the intriguing interaction between testosterone and neurocognitive development in males with 47,XXY. Curr Opin Obstet Gynecol 2020;32(2):140–6.
40. Samango-Sprouse C, Counts D, Gropman A, Focus Foundation. Insight versus hindsight: What we have learned after 17 years of research with sex chromosome abnormalities. Am J Med Genet 2021;185(3):1004–5.
41. Samango-Sprouse CA, Sadeghin T, Mitchell FL, et al. Positive effects of short course androgen therapy on the neurodevelopmental outcome in boys with 47,XXY syndrome at 36 and 72 months of age. Am J Med Genet 2013;161A(3): 501–8.
42. Samango-Sprouse C, Brooks MR, Counts D, et al. A longitudinal perspective of hormone replacement therapies (HRTs) on neuromotor capabilities in males with 47,XXY (Klinefelter syndrome). Genet Med 2022;24(6):1274–82.
43. Tran SL, Samango-Sprouse CA, Sadeghin T, et al. Hormonal replacement therapy and its potential influence on working memory and competency/adaptive functioning in 47,XXY (Klinefelter syndrome). Am J Med Genet 2019;179(12): 2374–81.
44. Foland-Ross LC, Ross JL, Reiss AL. Androgen treatment effects on hippocampus structure in boys with Klinefelter syndrome. Psychoneuroendocrinology 2019; 100:223–8.

45. Ross JL, Kushner H, Kowal K, et al. Androgen Treatment Effects on Motor Function, Cognition, and Behavior in Boys with Klinefelter Syndrome. J Pediatr 2017; 185:193–9.e4.

46. Hamzik MP, Gropman AL, Brooks MR, et al. The Effect of Hormonal Therapy on the Behavioral Outcomes in 47,XXY (Klinefelter Syndrome) between 7 and 12 Years of Age. Genes 2023;14(7):1402.

47. Samango-Sprouse C, Stapleton EJ, Lawson P, et al. Positive effects of early androgen therapy on the behavioral phenotype of boys with 47,XXY. Am J Med Genet C Semin Med Genet 2015;169(2):150–7.

48. Gravholt CH, Jensen AS, Høst C, et al. Body composition, metabolic syndrome and type 2 diabetes in Klinefelter syndrome. Acta Paediatr 2011;100(6):871–7.

49. Swerdlow AJ, Higgins CD, Schoemaker MJ, et al, United Kingdom Clinical Cytogenetics Group. Mortality in patients with Klinefelter syndrome in Britain: a cohort study. J Clin Endocrinol Metab 2005;90(12):6516–22.

50. Davis SM, Cox-Martin MG, Bardsley MZ, et al. Effects of Oxandrolone on Cardiometabolic Health in Boys With Klinefelter Syndrome: A Randomized Controlled Trial. J Clin Endocrinol Metab 2017;102(1):176–84.

51. Traish AM, Haider A, Doros G, et al. Long-term testosterone therapy in hypogonadal men ameliorates elements of the metabolic syndrome: an observational, long-term registry study. Int J Clin Pract 2014;68(3):314–29.

52. Davis S, Lahlou N, Bardsley M, et al. Gonadal function is associated with cardiometabolic health in pre-pubertal boys with Klinefelter syndrome. Andrology 2016;4(6):1169–77.

53. Ferlin A, Schipilliti M, Di Mambro A, et al. Osteoporosis in Klinefelter's syndrome. Mol Hum Reprod 2010;16(6):402–10.

54. Pizzocaro A, Vena W, Condorelli R, et al. Testosterone treatment in male patients with Klinefelter syndrome: a systematic review and meta-analysis. J Endocrinol Invest 2020;43(12):1675–87.

55. Vanderschueren D, Laurent MR, Claessens F, et al. Sex steroid actions in male bone. Endocr Rev 2014;35(6):906–60.

56. Bi LX, Wiren KM, Zhang XW, et al. The effect of oxandrolone treatment on human osteoblastic cells. J Burns Wounds 2007;6:e4.

57. Vogiatzi MG, Davis SM, Ross JL. Cortical Bone Mass is Low in Boys with Klinefelter Syndrome and Improves with Oxandrolone. J Endocr Soc 2021;5(4): bvab016.

58. Davis SM, Lahlou N, Cox-Martin M, et al. Oxandrolone Treatment Results in an Increased Risk of Gonadarche in Prepubertal Boys With Klinefelter Syndrome. J Clin Endocrinol Metab 2018;103(9):3449–55.

59. Courant F, Aksglaede L, Antignac JP, et al. Assessment of circulating sex steroid levels in prepubertal and pubertal boys and girls by a novel ultrasensitive gas chromatography-tandem mass spectrometry method. J Clin Endocrinol Metab 2010;95(1):82–92.

60. Apter D, Lenko HL, Perheentupa J, et al. Subnormal pubertal increases of serum androgens in Turner's syndrome. Horm Res 1982;16(3):164–73.

61. Ross JL, Quigley CA, Cao D, et al. Growth hormone plus childhood low-dose estrogen in Turner's syndrome. N Engl J Med 2011;364(13):1230–42.

62. Bareille P, Massarano AA, Stanhope R. Final height outcome in girls with Turner syndrome treated with a combination of low dose oestrogen and oxandrolone. Eur J Pediatr 1997;156(5):358–62.

63. Quigley CA, Crowe BJ, Anglin DG, et al. Growth hormone and low dose estrogen in Turner syndrome: results of a United States multi-center trial to near-final height. J Clin Endocrinol Metab 2002;87(5):2033–41.
64. Carel JC, Elie C, Ecosse E, et al. Self-esteem and social adjustment in young women with Turner syndrome–influence of pubertal management and sexuality: population-based cohort study. J Clin Endocrinol Metab 2006;91(8):2972–9.
65. Ruszala A, Wojcik M, Zygmunt-Gorska A, et al. Prepubertal ultra-low-dose estrogen therapy is associated with healthier lipid profile than conventional estrogen replacement for pubertal induction in adolescent girls with Turner syndrome: preliminary results. J Endocrinol Invest 2017;40(8):875–9.
66. Hasegawa Y, Ariyasu D, Izawa M, et al. Gradually increasing ethinyl estradiol for Turner syndrome may produce good final height but not ideal BMD. Endocr J 2017;64(2):221–7.
67. Ross JL, Roeltgen D, Feuillan P, et al. Use of estrogen in young girls with Turner syndrome: effects on memory. Neurology 2000;54(1):164–70.
68. Gravholt CH, Andersen NH, Conway GS, et al. Clinical practice guidelines for the care of girls and women with Turner syndrome: proceedings from the 2016 Cincinnati International Turner Syndrome Meeting. Eur J Endocrinol 2017;177(3): G1–70.

Moving?

Make sure your subscription moves with you!

To notify us of your new address, find your **Clinics Account Number** (located on your mailing label above your name), and contact customer service at:

Email: journalscustomerservice-usa@elsevier.com

800-654-2452 (subscribers in the U.S. & Canada)
314-447-8871 (subscribers outside of the U.S. & Canada)

Fax number: 314-447-8029

Elsevier Health Sciences Division
Subscription Customer Service
3251 Riverport Lane
Maryland Heights, MO 63043

*To ensure uninterrupted delivery of your subscription, please notify us at least 4 weeks in advance of move.

Printed and bound by CPI Group (UK) Ltd, Croydon, CR0 4YY

08/05/2025

01864724-0009